Praise for

LIFTED

Starting your day with Holly is not only a great workout, but a blast of positive energy to get you thru your day and feeling good! She truly is one of the BEST in her field!

—**Josh Capon, celebrity chef**

This book includes all the good energy and (non-cheesy) life-changing inspiration that Holly delivers on the bike and in her workouts that's made her one of the most deserving stars of the booming boutique fitness scene. One chapter = 1 workout!

Everyone needs Holly's feel-good ethos and coaching in their life. Read this if you've ever wondered how to have more legitimate happiness—and wondered why workouts and clean eating alone haven't gotten you there. The inner life plan Holly shares taps the latest information about the power of fitness and meditation to transform your life in a way that's science-supported, incredibly fun, empowering, and realistic.

Holly is a real-deal fitness rock star who's built a passionate following by tapping into what she knows can help empower and even heal people. She is a powerful voice in the new fitness generation.

—**Melisse Gelula, cofounder of Well+Good**

Holly is changing my life one class at a time! Her combination of genuine charisma, mindful technique, and expert guidance makes her my favorite instructor on the planet, and LIFTED is the only class I refuse to miss.

—**Isaac Hindin-Miller, writer**

Holly Rilinger is brilliant in designing a complete lifestyle program, combining the time-tested principles of mental focus, mobility, strength-building exercises, and spiritual elevation.

Having been Holly's college strength and conditioning coach, I saw first-hand her desire for knowledge in human performance. It was revealed in college that she had a natural propensity for helping others and being a team leader. I'm so happy to see she has followed her heart and has grown into a world-class trainer, and I'm even more happy to see how she has dedicated her life's work to helping others reach their human performance goals.

LIFTED is a program that can benefit everyone, from the beginner who's on a quest to become healthier to the person who's followed a traditional fitness program for years and needs a deeper connection to their why's of complete human performance. I have been in the human performance industry for more than thirty years and today I got started on LIFTED!

—Coach Greg Werner

LIFTED

---

28 DAYS TO

STRENGTHEN YOUR BODY

FOCUS YOUR MIND + ELEVATE YOUR SPIRIT

HOLLY RILINGER

WITH MYATT MURPHY

Da Capo

LIFE
LONG

Copyright © 2017 by Holly Rilinger
Interior photographs by Matt Doyle

Editorial production by Lori Hobkirk at the Book Factory
Interior book design by Cynthia Young
Set in 11.75 point Adobe Garamond

Cataloging-in-Publication data for this book is available from the Library of Congress.
First Da Capo Press edition 2017
ISBN: 978-0-7382-1994-3 (paperback)
ISBN: 978-0-7382-1995-0 (e-book)

Published by Da Capo Press, an imprint of Perseus Books,
a subsidiary of Hachette Books Group, Inc.
www.dacapopress.com

Note: The information in this book is true and complete to the best of our knowledge. This book is intended only as an informative guide for those wishing to know more about health issues. In no way is this book intended to replace, countermand, or conflict with the advice given to you by your own physician. The ultimate decision concerning care should be made between you and your doctor. We strongly recommend you follow his or her advice. Information in this book is general and is offered with no guarantees on the part of the authors or Da Capo Press. The authors and publisher disclaim all liability in connection with the use of this book.

Da Capo Press books are available at special discounts for bulk purchases in the United States by corporations, institutions, and other organizations. For more information, please contact the Special Markets Department at the Perseus Books Group, 2300 Chestnut Street, Suite 200, Philadelphia, PA 19103, or call (800) 810-4145, ext. 5000, or e-mail special.markets@perseusbooks.com.19103, or call (800) 810-4145, ext. 5000, or e-mail special.markets@perseusbooks.com.

10 9 8 7 6 5 4 3 2 1

Dedicated to all of you and the greatness inside of you—
find your wings and fly.

Most of all to my family.
Thank you for your undying love,
your support, and your sacrifice.
I love you all.

Contents

Introduction

Why are you reading this book? In other words, *why* do you want to try LIFTED?

Maybe you think it's obvious. I mean, there are a million infomercials out there tempting us to buy something so we can have what we think we want or need. So maybe your *why* is to have

The perfect butt!

Sexy six pack!

Legs of steel!

Don't get me wrong—that's all very enticing. After all, who doesn't want to have an amazing, sexy, and strong body? In fact, most people's *why* is rooted in their bodies, and I don't see anything wrong with wanting these things.

However, if these are the only things that fuel your journey, you'll eventually fall short. No matter how much you exercise, you'll never be satisfied and never find joy—even if you get in the best shape of your life—if you don't discover your *why* and rethink it. Most programs don't focus on the real reason why you may want to lose weight in the first place. It's why so many people crash and burn on the fat-loss programs they try: they focus only on losing pounds, and even if they manage to succeed, they go right back to what they were doing. That's because they may address "weight loss," but they never address the *why*. You need to trace back to *WHY* you would want to have the perfect butt, sexy six-pack abs, or legs of steel—or all three!

When I ask clients *why* they want to change their appearance and keep asking them over and over again, eventually—I get to their real *why*.

Why? *Because I'll look hot!*

Why is that important? *Looking hot means people will think I'm sexy!*

Why is that important? *Being sexy means I'll get attention.*

Why is that important? *Attention will lead to finding a special person.*

Why is that important? *That special person will offer me love.*

AND THERE IT IS. *Love.*

At the end of the day most of the things we want and need all point back to finding love and being happier. In my classes I hear more people than ever tell me they want to feel happy and live without stress. But they are also still rooted in believing the best way to get there is through having perfect abs, a rock-hard body, and looking better in their clothes.

They rarely think about the mind or the spirit. Because even if an exercise program works for you and you reach your target weight, if you haven't addressed *why* you want to lose weight in the first place, you may not be satisfied with the results.

You're ignoring the underlying current that's going to create consistency, longevity, and real happiness. Which is why you'll continue to fall back to that unhappy place. You will inevitably have bad days. You might give up. Until the next time you see a pair of jeans or feel pressure about summer, or your wedding, and decide you want to be in shape again.

THE REASON LIFTED WORKS so well is that it provides a solution to that yo-yo approach by encouraging you to tap into things beyond the body. Over the next twenty-eight days you'll be following a different path to get you over your fitness hurdles, make new habits, and change your life. But it will take going out of your old comfort zones to get there.

If you're ready to trade your comfort in for change, I guarantee we'll get there together. You're looking for someone to help you along the way. And guess what—you found her.

WHO AM I? I'm currently the creative director at Cyc Fitness and was a founding instructor at Flywheel, where for six years I had thousands of people walk through the door. Three years ago I joined forces with Nike as a master trainer and currently mentor Nike's East Coast team of trainers. I've also built my own business from the ground up and have traveled the globe hosting destination camps, speaking to people of all ages, and inspiring change one person at a time.

NOW THERE ARE a lot of people who look at elite trainers and think, *How do you know what I feel? You've probably never been fat a day in your life.* And maybe you're thinking something like that right now. Maybe you've come to believe it's impossible to lose weight, get fit, and have a richer, happier life—and you have doubts that I can help you make that happen because I couldn't possibly understand what you're feeling and the challenges you face.

But if there's one thing I know about, it's what it feels like to have a dream that the rest of the world thinks is impossible.

I had decided when I was six years old that I would play professional basketball one day. Even though there wasn't a pro league for women at that time. Even though I was short and would grow up to be only five-feet-four.

I had all odds stacked against me. But I spent the next fifteen years turning my dream into a reality, and eventually I played pro basketball for five years.

What I didn't realize at the time was that I was teaching myself how to be a coach. I wasn't born a great basketball player destined to go pro; it took tens of thousands of hours of hard work, training my mind, body, and spirit. And without all three I never would have accomplished everything I did. Mastering how to motivate myself helped me become one of the best motivators in the game, and my passion for basketball eventually evolved into a new life's work: helping others get the body of their dreams and leading them to the life they've always wanted. And as many twists and turns as my career has taken, that three-part approach to training mind, body, and spirit has remained at the core of my philosophy—and I know it can work for you too.

When I first launched my LIFTED class—a new method that incorporates meditation and spirituality with high-intensity exercise—it was incredible to watch how well it was received and how successful it's now become. LIFTED may be an intense training program, but it brings in elements that are far from intense and what's missing in most programs—both tranquility and spirituality.

You see, my philosophy is to bring the mind, body, and spirit together into one single workout. You owe it to yourself to channel all three into everything you do. If you have a deficit in any of those three areas, you're not going to have a complete workout. You're not going to be a complete person.

You're not going to have a complete life.

When you're not happy with your body, it brings down your spirit. When you have too much on your mind, that stress can cause your body to store fat. When your spirit's down, you may make unhealthier lifestyle and nutritional choices that keep you from moving forward. And these are just a few ways all three affect each other.

You can't separate them, so doesn't it make sense to embark on a program that brings the three together?

I knew early on that all three things needed to be present, and I watched all three work together in my career and my life. I watched all three create this little whirlwind that became more and more powerful. But when I take one out, that whirlwind becomes lopsided and stops spinning upward.

It goes from LIFTing you up to holding you down.

I've had plenty of people tell me they rarely feel joy when they work out. But if you're open to experiencing what exercise could be—what happens when you make working out a complete mind, body, and spirit experience—then you'll be more likely to experience that joy, reach your goals, realize your dreams . . . and LIFT your life.

OVER THE TWENTY-EIGHT DAYS of the LIFTED program, the role I'll play in your life is one of a coach, yes, but also as a teammate.

I'll be shoulder to shoulder with you, sweating alongside you, and your victories will be *our* victories. This is what I want for you, and I can get you there. I want you to be the type of person who wakes up on fire, follows their light, and lives in their truth. The type who falls down, skins their knees, and gets right back up. I want you to dream your biggest dream and fall in love with your life every day.

What I want for you is the best life you can possibly live, and it would be my honor to help you find it. As long as you're willing to stop looking for happiness in the same place you lost it and realize that what is coming is better than what is gone, we can do it—you and me.

So what's *my why*?

It used to be basketball—but now it's you.

Right now, my *why* is to LIFT as many people as possible by getting them to understand what I've learned along the way and what has worked for not just me but the lives of everyone I've been lucky enough to train and teach over the years.

My entire mission in life is to LIFT.

That's why I do it.

You're why I do it.

So let's do it together!

—Holly

Finding Your Why

I have aspirations just like anyone else, and those aspirations helped me become one of the top trainers in the fitness industry. It took courage and confidence. It involved taking risks and being vulnerable. And it required a daily energy, even on days when I didn't have it. And I'll be honest: for a long time I didn't know my true *why*.

Yet there was something there. I could feel it.

Basketball was a no-brainer, but it took a little digging to understand why I was doing this fitness thing. Sure, I had been training my whole life, but was there heart in this for me? When I dug deep and really tried to figure out why sharing what I know about fitness and exercise was so important, it finally made sense.

Knowing my *why* makes all things possible. It's there for me when I wake up in the morning and see all the things that I have to do that day. It's there for me when I look at the entire staircase instead of just the first step and suddenly feel incredibly overwhelmed. It's because of my *why* that I know that if I do the things I'm preaching about, if I take my own advice about meditation and exercise and doing the things to LIFT my spirit, I can tackle it all.

Knowing my *why* makes the things I need to do along the way far more manageable and enjoyable. Because I'm constantly reminded that each thing I'm doing for my mind, body, and spirit is bringing me closer to the reason *why* I'm doing everything in the first place.

Even though you need to figure out what your *why* is, if you don't know what it is yet, that's okay. Because I can guarantee that your actual *why* is not a size-four jeans.

Mindfulness is a huge component of LIFTED, and it permeates throughout every portion of the program. You might find your *why* in a quiet moment as you meditate. It may come to you at the end of one of the workouts. It may happen when you perform something I ask you to do to LIFT your spirit.

The truth is, if you're not very spiritually minded at the start, finding your *why* may be the hardest thing to do in this book. But as you move through the LIFTED program you'll begin to do things that will open your mind and spirit to new possibilities and experiences. Your *why* will begin to come more into focus as LIFTED makes you more honest with yourself.

So even though you may not be able to initially connect with it yet, as you go through the program—I promise—you will find your why.

In fact, you may find several.

Or you may think you have your *why* right now, only to discover that as you open up, your *why* may change.

But you will find it. It might not necessarily be some epiphany where the skies part—but you'll find it.

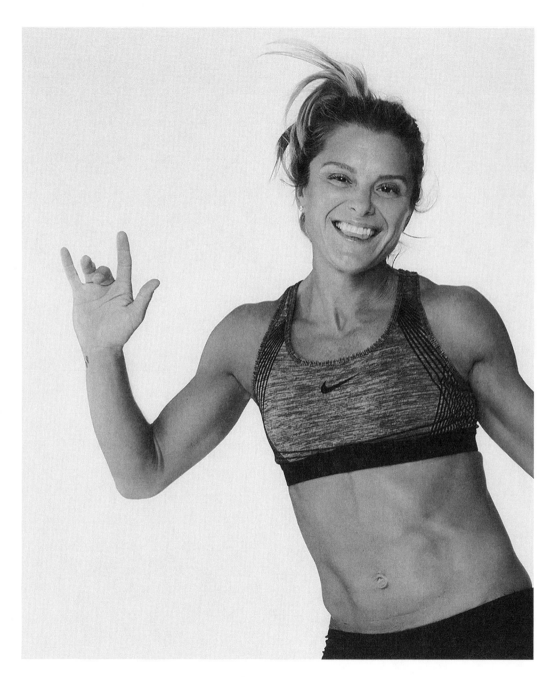

THE BASICS

1

Why Do You Really
Want to Fly?

Before LIFTED can help you fly, you need to decide where you want it to take you.

I believe most people have an overall sense of a "feeling" they want to arrive at when they take on a lifestyle program to lose weight and change their life. But when I ask people online or in my class what their goal is for the weekend or dig even deeper and ask what their one-year goal is for themselves, I'm always hit with the same vague replies.

For example, people love to tell me that they want to be fit, but that's not a goal—that's a feeling that could be measured in many different ways. The same goes for wanting to be leaner, healthier, or stronger. It's great to *want* to be all these things, but they're not anything you can technically check off your list because they're not specific and measurable.

Draw It Up—Then Dream

You've gotta dream and imagine your perfect life, but know this: a dream without a plan is nothing more than a wish.

If I had simply closed my eyes and imagined that I had basketball skills, I would never have—could never have—played professional basketball. I had to come face to face with my dreams on a daily basis. I had to sit down and ask myself what I really wanted in life. I needed to think about what goals I had to achieve in the short and long term to move closer to my dreams.

I had to design my life—the life I wanted to have.

I had to make daily sacrifices and show up even when I didn't feel like it.

If that sounds daunting to you, I promise it's not as complicated as it sounds. But the fact remains: you can't move forward if you don't know which direction you should go, and a person without a goal is like a ship without a sail.

That's *not* going to be you. I'm going to show you how to work the program, and I'm here to give you the tools you need.

Get Your Goals in Gear!

I'm a big believer in taking the time to break things out into one-year, five-year, and ten-year goals. And I will admit, the first time I thought this way I felt so much pressure. I couldn't imagine thinking that far ahead, even though I had technically done that as a kid when it came to wanting to play basketball—then it was easy for me!

But remember, as children we feel uninhibited and unphased by the things that may deflate our dreams. That's why you need to turn back time and start using the mind you used to dream with as a child.

It's time to set up goals of your own. What I want you to do is think about and write down two types of goals: outcome and process.

Outcome Goals

Outcome goals are the goals you're hoping to achieve. They need to be definable. You can't just say you want to be fit—you need to hone in on what you wish to be fit for. You can't just say you want to lose weight—you should know how much weight you would like to lose. You shouldn't just say you want to eat healthier—you should know exactly what types of foods you want to eat more of and which type of foods you want to eat less of.

For example:

- I will lower my blood pressure by twenty points.
- I will lose five pounds.
- I will double how many veggies I eat each week.

Notice I used the words "I will." You need to *believe* your goals from the moment they make their way to paper.

Process Goals

Process goals are the goals you have to hit in order to make your outcome goals a reality. They are the tangible goals—the ones that you can actually do. These are the goals that get you where you want to go and make your outcome goals reachable. They need to be things that at the end of the week you can reflect back on and say, "According to what I said I'd do and what I actually did, either this week brought me closer to where I want to be—or it didn't."

For example:

- I will meditate for at least ten minutes a day.
- I will work out four times per week.
- I will make my lunch and dinner three-fourths veggies every meal.

So . . . why both?

I love to talk to children about this because when you sit in front of a bunch of young athletes and ask how many of them want to be pro athletes, every single hand goes up.

I get it. Who doesn't? You're looking at a future that comes off like a big shiny toy—flying in private jets, having world fame, making lots of money. There aren't too many people on the planet who wouldn't want that to happen.

That's because most people have outcome goals. But they either don't have process goals in place or don't want to have them. Because then there's more of a commitment to take action instead of hoping good things will come our way without having to try so hard. It's all about wishing and not about working toward that wish. After all, when it comes down to it, accomplishing big goals means big sacrifices and commitment.

There are other people who focus only on process goals but never have an outcome goal. Have you ever seen that person who continuously works out and never seems happy? Ever met a workaholic who can't seem to stop for a moment to appreciate what they have? That's a person without an outcome goal. These people become so absorbed in the process that they never take the time to define "What's the ideal weight I want to be?" or "How much money is enough?" So they keep going, never satisfying their spirit because their goals are never in balance with one another.

That's why you need both to make your dreams come true. Your outcome goals are the destination—they are your *I wants*. Your process goals are the journey—they are your *I wills*.

So . . . write them down!

For the sake of the LIFTED program I want your goals to be related to what you think my program can help you achieve. I also want your goals to be realistic and measurable within the four weeks you'll be using the program. Putting down that you want to lose fifty pounds in four weeks isn't going to happen because it's impossible, so stick with outcome goals that are attainable.

I also don't want anything to ever be a number that overwhelms you. I find that if I ask clients to write too many goals, sometimes they stretch their goals out too thin. Instead, I've found that sticking with three outcome goals is fairly reasonable. You can always have more, but three is a great starting point. Let's set ourselves up for a VICTORY!

As for choosing your process goals, I'll be taking care of that for you. That's the beauty of LIFTED. Simply by following the four-week program you'll be lifting your mind, body, and spirit, which I guarantee will put you down the path of achieving your outcome goals. So for now these will be your process goals:

- I will do all the prescribed workouts for the entire four weeks.
- I will meditate every single morning.
- I will check in with my Dream Board every day (don't worry—I'll explain that one later in the chapter).
- I will visualize a minimum of twice a day (don't worry—I'm about to explain this one right now!).

It's in YOU—I know it.

People tend to believe that greatness is reserved for the elite, but greatness is in all of us.

Oftentimes when we're unsure of our personal path, we look at other people's accomplishments and compare ourselves to them. We look at the things others are doing, question our potential, and doubt that the same greatness is inside of us. But as it's said, "You should never compare your first chapter to someone else's twentieth chapter."

Many of the people we admire also had the same humble beginnings you may be having right now. They had the same fears and setbacks. The only reason you're seeing them where they are now—at their most successful position in life—is that they persevered.

I thought that when I first started training in New York. I wondered how I could ever compete in such a huge city. But it starts with a seed. And what fertilizes that seed is recognizing that greatness is in you—it's just that you need to nurture and cultivate each tiny seed.

No one else can do that for you. My parents couldn't force me to practice or train. No coach could make me the player I was. No one could push me as far as I could push myself. It's as simple as starting with a belief and having a little faith in yourself.

Visualization: See It and Free It!

When I was a kid I was driven purely by passion. And at that time I developed certain skills around that passion that I had no idea were actually tools that have been proven to enhance performance. One of those skills was visualization.

At night I would lie on my bed, close my eyes, and clearly visualize myself on the court. I could see myself dribbling down the court effortlessly and pulling up for a jump shot. I could feel the ball in my hands, notice my breath, and hear the crowd hush—and then *erupt*! I would do it to the point where my muscles would twitch, where it felt as if I were actually doing it, even though I was only doing it in my head. It felt so real, I would have to stop because I couldn't sleep. Innately I did this as a kid because it was exciting. But the best athletes in the world rely on this technique because they know the body will do whatever the mind believes it can do. They understand that once your mind has conceived something—the body naturally has an easier time doing it.

For example, when researchers in France studied the effect of visualization on high jumpers, their performance improved by 35 percent.[1] Better still, by adding in physical movements as they visualized—for example, by mimicking simple arm movements—they managed to raise their performance up to 45 percent. It turns out that what I was doing as a little girl—just closing my eyes, holding a ball in my hands in my bed, and thinking through the motions—is something now backed by science.

Fast forward to today, and I still use visualization; it's been a constant tool for my entire life. As an instructor I'm no longer performance based, but to this day I'll have certain spin classes where I might be nervous, don't feel I'm on my game, or might be just a little bit depleted from life. Yet I have to go in and motivate sixty other people.

That's when I use visualization to make my thoughts connect to my body so I can produce the state and results I want to have in every class.

The power of visualization is underrated and often overlooked, yet it's one of the most powerful tools you can add to your toolbox.

Make it work for you as you use LIFTED.

Picture Every Part of Yourself

The magic of LIFTED is that the program affects every part of your life—mind, body, and spirit. So when you visualize, there are no limits.

If you have an interview the next day, close your eyes and imagine yourself feeling confident, stepping into the room tall, and making eye contact with everybody. Picture yourself having a very fluid conversation in which you're articulate and have an answer for every question they ask.

If you have a race the next day or just a training session, close your eyes and think about running every step or going through every motion. Let yourself feel what it will be like when you cross the finish line or complete the class. Imagine every part of it being effortless and enjoyable.

But know this: you don't have to save visualization for special occasions or events; we always have something to do the next day that we could do a little better. So whatever that might be, so long as it's important to you to do your best, incorporating visualization can benefit you.

Picture a Perfect Performance

As you visualize, failure is not an option. Some people will imagine themselves doing something and find themselves automatically thinking about how they might trip themselves up along the way. That is not what I want you to do. Your body can hear what you are thinking and saying about it. For real. So you need to choose your thoughts and words carefully.

It's important to forget about any flaws. Visualization sets the stage for how you feel and what amount of energy you take into whatever it is you're visualizing. So all you should be picturing is your perfect self. You need to imagine that whatever you're doing, you're not only doing it perfectly but effortlessly as well.

A recent UK study involving more than forty-four thousand subjects found that just by imagining you can do a specific task better, that's exactly what happens as a result.[2] When researchers measured the effects of various motivational methods, the greatest improvements to performance came either when subjects told themselves out loud that they could beat their best score or react faster or when they imagined they could beat their best score or react faster.

That's why three-quarters through my class I will tell people that they have a choice at that moment. They can perceive themselves as exhausted, or they can perceive themselves as exhilarated. One of those choices will make that experience far easier and more enjoyable than the other one. It's your choice—only when your mind is your ally will you actually begin to see change.

Close Your Eyes Often

Checking visualization off your list each day is pretty easy to do, but for now all I want you to do is try it for a couple of minutes twice a day.

It can be at your desk. It can be on the subway or the bus. It can be while you're waiting for your kids or waiting for your coffee to brew. Eventually you may find yourself doing it fifteen to twenty times a day, and that's okay! The more you picture yourself performing in your prime, the more you'll believe you can—and the more likely you will. Remember: children daydream all day long. Somewhere along the way as adults we tend to lose this—GET IT BACK!

Some of my favorite times to do it are

In the morning: I always recommend doing some visualization in the morning because mornings are always a fresh start to everything. After all, if you can visualize the perfect day, just think about how much better the rest of your day will be.

The night before anything big: As much as I love the mornings, there are typically a lot of things that could easily distract me from doing it the morning of a big event. That's when I'll do it the night before, right before bedtime.

Any time! It takes only a few seconds to bring yourself back into the space of confidence that visualization creates—so don't be afraid to try it anywhere at any time.

I would visualize in the middle of a basketball game at the free throw line. I had a ritual every single time. My right foot would be on the line. The referee would bounce the ball to me. It would come into my hands, and I would immediately close my eyes. And for two seconds I would see the ball go through the net. I would then dribble the ball three times, bend my knees, and get ready to shoot, and I would watch the ball roll off my fingers and—go through the net.

You could be in the middle of an exercise class, know that a hard part was about to come up, then close your eyes and imagine yourself doing it perfectly. You could be seconds away from being introduced to give a speech and look down, close your eyes, and imagine yourself striding up to the podium, looking confident and strong.

So just remember: even in crunch time, when you think you don't have a moment, there's always a few seconds to spare.

Make It a Sensory Experience

It's not just about imagining yourself doing something perfectly; it's also about imagining exactly how that moment will feel from every possible perspective. Bringing as many elements into your moment—the little things that might be happening behind the scenes—adds to the experience and makes it more powerful.

The more detail you can bring into your visualization, the more real it will feel. So as you're visualizing, try walking yourself through all five senses if possible.

Visualize the Perfect Meal

If eating is an area of weakness for you, then using visualization as a tool to help you make better choices can have a powerful effect. Believe it or not, if you just close your eyes before taking your first bite to imagine eating healthy, you're less likely to run into surprises and can deflect them when they come.

This can especially be helpful when dining out with friends where you may not have as much willpower. Take the time to picture yourself saying no to the breadbasket. Imagine yourself having only one drink. Allow yourself to feel incredibly confident with every decision you make instead of worrying about what other people may think of your decisions.

By visualizing it first, you'll be able to recognize that the reactions you *thought* people might have to your decisions never occur. Many times it's that split-second yes or no that gets us in trouble with food. But through visualization you have that time to think about how you would react and what the better choices might be in that moment, so you're more prepared to make those smarter choices when you actually have that meal. That way, once you step into that meal, it's like reliving that moment all over again— and you'll have an easier time saying no to any unhealthy eats.

- What would you be hearing at that moment?
- What would you be seeing in front of you—and all around you?
- What would you feel under your feet, in your hands, or any place from head to toe?
- Would you smell fresh-cut grass as you ran a race, or would you smell the leather seats in the boardroom where you had to give a presentation?

The more real you can make it, the more you'll actually feel like you've done it!

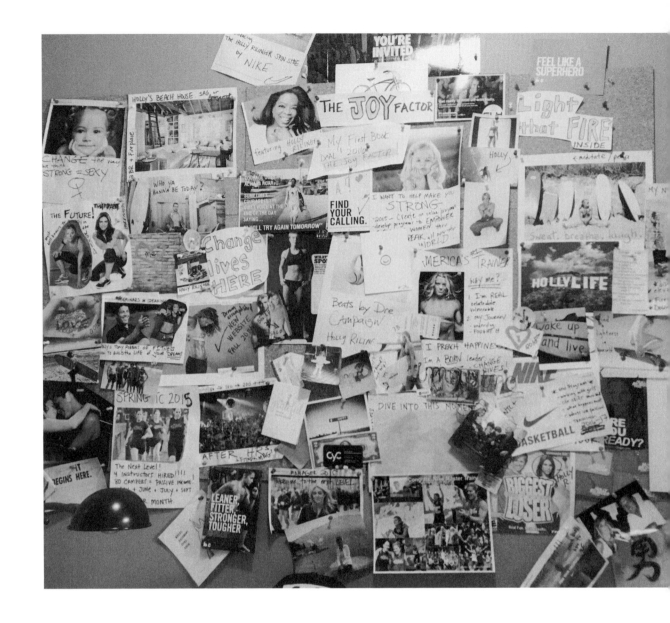

Your Dream Board

As a child I would plaster my room, from window to wall, with pictures and posters of the players I admired. So when you stepped into my room, you stepped into my dreams, and instantly you would feel what I was all about. This is another powerful visualization technique I've been using for longer than I realized.

I only did it because it made perfect sense to me: Why wouldn't I want to look at my heroes the first thing in the morning? Because it incites passion in me—it sparked a fire. Even on days when it was raining or I felt too tired to start the day, I would see those photos and be reminded of exactly why it made sense for me to get up and continue to chase my dreams.

I still use this technique to aid in visualization in the form of my Dream Board.

Tucked in a little nook by my desk where I have my morning coffee is a bulletin board filled with cut out pictures, pieces of paper with writing on them, and other objects. And each represents a dream. That way, when I wake up I always come face-to-face with my current dreams. I'm reminded each morning what drives me, what inspires me, what I'm passionate about, and, most importantly, what my focus is.

My Dream Board is my perfect painting of the way I want my life to play out. And now I'm sharing that with you.

It doesn't take much. Mine is a very seasoned Dream Board now, but when I first put it up, it might've had five things on it at most. Now it takes up an entire wall, with pictures and pieces of paper orbiting all the way around the bulletin board hidden underneath.

If I had to count, there are probably fifty to sixty dreams on it—a mix of short-term dreams, long-term dreams, laughable dreams, and dreams that once seemed impossible at one time, but yet I managed to make them happen. In fact, while working on this portion of the book I spent a little extra time looking at my Dream Board and surprised myself to see a piece of paper up there that said these little words: *My first book deal. 2016!*

My point: this book started as nothing more than a dream. It began as a single piece of paper tacked up on my Dream Board. And seeing it every single day, along with setting goals and using the power of visualization, made it happen. It's time you face your dreams so they can inspire you to help make them come true.

But know this: the rules are . . . there are no rules!

I believe your Dream Board should be like a piece of art. I honestly feel it should be different for every single person. So I could tell you how to create it precisely, but that might not work for you. After all, they are your dreams, not mine.

I would never give you too many restrictions because I would never limit your dreams. I would also never tell you what to dream. But there are a few guidelines that can help you get started.

Find a Space That Speaks to You

You don't need an actual bulletin board. It can just be a blank wall. It can be your refrigerator. It can be whatever is the best place for you to hang your dreams so you never miss looking at them every single day.

Start with Six—But Mix!

Your Dream Board should be a lawless territory, and I would never tell you how many dreams to have. But to give you a nice baseline, try to start with at least six dreams—three short-term and three long-term dreams. Just be sure they're *not* all tied into one specific thing, such as weight loss.

If your dreams are only one dimensional, you'll be moving in only one direction. I want you to be growing in all directions, and the only way to do that is to make sure you dream outside the box.

For me, I have a lot of work-related dreams, but I also have a lot of play-related dreams, such as places I want to travel to or even something as simple as a Broadway show I want to see one day. I also have love and relationship dreams, along with short- and long-term lifestyle dreams. And yes, I also have body dreams too—just like you. So make a point of looking at all the things you wish to change in your life, and if possible, make sure there's at least one dream up there that speaks to each.

Dare to Dream the Impossible

A lot of people will tell you to set realistic dreams, but I have mixed feelings about that. Because I believe that if people aren't laughing at your dreams, then they probably aren't big enough.

My very first dream was being a professional basketball player. But here's something you might not know. Back when I was a little girl there wasn't a professional basketball league for women. My dream didn't even exist yet! But that never stopped me from dreaming the impossible. There was never a moment when I ever thought I couldn't do it.

As I got older I've had moments in life when I've started to doubt myself. I've had those moments when the things I hoped to achieve seemed less possible. But I also found a way to carry that youthful, invincible feeling through life with me and continuously tap into making the impossible possible. I knew that as long as I could back up my dreams with passion and a plan, any of them could become a reality.

So if you think what you're passionate about is impossible, if you think others will laugh at your dream, then know you're doing it right. A lot of times we limit our dreams based on what other people will think about us. So forget about them—get out there and make them all laugh.

Recognize the Power of Pictures

I feel pictures are way more powerful than words, but I also feel that you need to be as specific as possible with your dreams. If you're not specific about what you throw out there, you can't be sure about what's going to come back to you.

That said, if you're using pictures to describe your dreams, try to find pictures that depict as closely as possible what you hope to achieve. Once you have a picture, write on it exactly why you put it on your Dream Board. You can even go so far as to put a date on the picture, stating when you hope to achieve that dream. The more detailed you make it, the more you can expect it to come true.

Put What Matters Most in the Middle

I place the dreams that are the most important to me right in the center of my board. It doesn't matter whether they're short- or long-term goals. What matters is that they are the dreams that make something jump inside me, even when I'm just thinking about them. The ones I feel are more pressing and passionate—those are the ones that move me the most.

Why dead center? It's human nature to look into the center of anything, and that's where my eyes go first every time. But it's so much more than that.

When we put them in the middle, they create an energy that can bring your Dream Board to life. I'll admit that at certain points along my journey I've had a few dreams I noticed were pinned on the outsides of my board—dreams I wanted to come true sooner than later. But when I moved them to the center, I truly felt as if I put energy into those dreams by physically changing where they were placed. And not surprisingly, it made a few of them come true.

If It No Longer Inspires—Retire It

Your heart should want everything on your Dream Board or be moved by it. But if anything isn't getting a reaction from your heart anymore, it might require a closer look and need to be taken down.

Sometimes there's an extra dream in our hearts we're not even thinking about until we have to. It sounds so simple, but taking time to remove what no longer speaks to you can free up a little more space and make you realize that you have a hole to fill.

The only time I don't want you to take something down from your Dream Board is because you think you cannot do it. It's okay to lose passion for something. It's okay to no longer want a dream. But if the reason you're reaching for that dream to remove is because you don't believe it will ever happen, then put that one right in the center.

Leave Up What You've Knocked Off

Just because you've accomplished a dream doesn't mean it has to come down. I have a few things up that I've accomplished. It's all part of being grateful.

I don't want you just reaching for things—I want you to remember what you've reached for and pulled into your world. Keeping up a few dreams you've crossed off your list will remind you of what was once a dream but is now a reality. It makes you believe that everything else that surrounds that accomplished dream can be accomplished too.

That also goes for things you've placed up there that aren't necessarily dreams but instead serve as inspiration. One of the things on my Dream Board is a set of four business cards. When I was first starting out and deciding on a logo for my business, I couldn't decide what color to choose—orange, blue, pink, or green—and those cards were the first time I was ever printing anything for myself business-wise. So I decided to go for all four colors! There's no relevance to them anymore, with the exception that they mark the beginning of where I am today, so I'm proud of them.

Follow a Feeling—And Find a New Dream

Not everything on your Dream Board has to be a dream. In fact, feel free to add a few things that simply move you in the moment. Once I put a picture of a surfer girl on my Dream Board because I just felt creative that day and loved that picture. When I realized I hadn't been very specific about why it was up there, I decided to write some questions on the picture: "The girl? The board? A surf trip?"

I wasn't necessarily clear on what I wanted from that picture, but there was something about it—so I put it up.

One year later, when I did a photo shoot for my rebrand, my agent brought up a photographer they wanted to shoot me, and it was the same person that had taken that picture on my Dream Board. (She's also the photographer I chose to shoot the cover of this book.)

Just by placing it on my board, I had put something out there. I had breathed life into that, even though I didn't know how that energy was going to come back to me. All I was clear about was that I wasn't sure. I was certain that the picture spoke to me, and my uncertainty didn't stop me from putting it up on my Dream Board.

So if something inspires you, even if you're not quite sure why, I want you to put it up there. There is a reason you are attracted to it and feel compelled to place it on your Dream Board. That means there could be something behind it—so don't let that opportunity pass.

It's Okay to Re-Date a Dream

I have certain dreams on my board that I swore I would accomplish by the date I wrote on them. But I'll admit it: I have a few up there that have one year crossed out and a later date scribbled on top. But I always remind myself—and I'm reminding you now—that things don't always happen within the time we expect them to. You can set a goal, and if it doesn't happen, you didn't fail—you just have to recalibrate!

Sprinkle in
Those Who Believe in Your Dreams

Throughout the years people have left me little notes telling me to keep going. Any pieces of encouragement that come your way are little blessings. They serve as reminders that there are other people who believe in you as much as you should believe in yourself.

That's why your Dream Board should also be a place where you collect these little pieces of encouragement. Each note or card or tiny gift pinned or taped up on your Dream Board brings momentum to your dreams.

So if someone ever gave you something that still has an impact on you today, don't tuck it away. Don't hide the energy those little things can bring to your life. Instead, let them add happiness and passion to your Dream Board. By placing them up there you're reminded of the people who believe in you, and this can help in those moments and on those days when you may not believe in yourself.

Finally . . . Duplicate Your Dreams

For many people it's a lot easier to set up a Dream Board in their house than somewhere else. But having it close by in a place that allows you to look at it constantly is key.

So if you have it set up where you live, take a picture of it and place it on your phone. Make it your screensaver on your computer, the wallpaper on your phone, or print it out and hang it someplace where you can always see it. That way, you'll always have the ability to look at it no matter where you are. It lets you take your dreams with you anywhere!

Get *LIFTED!*

So . . . you finally see that greatness is inside you—and you've wondered about your *why*. You've gathered all your goals, and you've displayed all your dreams. By now I think it's fairly obvious that this is no ordinary lifestyle program.

You see, working out isn't just about losing weight or getting stronger and fitter—it's practice for life. If everyone could understand that their workouts have the potential to make themselves better for everything else they do in life, we might not see the rates of chronic diseases related to sedentary lifestyles that we do today.

We would stop looking at exercise as a choice but rather as a necessity that positively affects every part of our day.

LIFTED—THE PROMISE

We all know people who blame something outside of themselves for their failures. That person who says things like, "Yoga doesn't work for me!" or "It's just genetics!" or "I'm doing what I'm supposed to do, and it doesn't work!"

But if these people would just stop, look at their life, and try to understand what they're putting out there that's being mirrored back to them, they would see the things they're not addressing in their lives.

By focusing on your mind, body, and spirit simultaneously, you give yourself the tools to figure out what's *really* behind what's holding you back, what you really want to do, and what really matters most.

Even though the main sections of the book are arranged in order of mind, body, and spirit, they aren't set up that way because that's how they're typically described. It's actually how my class flows—and how you'll flow through the program.

In my classes I start with the mind through meditation to open up my students to receive the class and help them surrender to the moment. We wash away all the distractions so we can perform better. We clean the slate.

Next we focus on the body through exercise (with a little more meditation in between), using a series of multimuscle movements that raise the heartbeat, activate more muscle fibers, and help make a stronger mind-muscle connection. And what happens at the end—what happens throughout—is a lifting of the spirit that they can bottle up and take with them throughout the day.

(Continues)

(Continued)

With LIFTED I'm not just giving you one angle of attack. I'm not just showing you how to engage all three when you work out. I'm not just showing you how to engage all three when you're not working out. I will show you how to engage all three from the second you wake up until the moment you fall asleep—and help get you excited about waking up each and every day to do it all over again!

LIFTED—THE LEAP

I understand that for some this journey might be a leap of faith. I know it might be a complete act of trust to take this little thing called fitness that you think is very ancillary and imagine that it can be done in a way that impacts you on every level. But if you believe what I am saying, that it has tentacles that can reach out and change your life, well, wouldn't that be amazing?

So what if I'm right?

What if this way of living that I'm about to show you not only transforms your body but also makes you happier, gives you more energy, and brings you a deeper sense of peace? What if it does all those things?

The fact that you're holding this book right now tells me there is a part of you that's willing to take that leap of faith. So know this:

Maybe you're thirty pounds overweight and don't have faith in yourself and don't believe you can do it. Maybe you're already in shape, but something's still missing in yourself. It doesn't matter. With LIFTED you're going to tap into that place that helped a five-foot-four kid become a pro athlete. This book is going to light that fire inside of you and turn you into your best coach and biggest fan. You will become that person who never wants to let you down and, from this point forward, never will.

I can give you this because I have cried it. I have sweat it. I have rejoiced in it. I have experienced it in my mind, body, and soul. So I can come to you and help you do the same thing.

This four-week program is a bridge that extends from how you think right now over to my way of thinking and a new lease on life. Turn this page, and you'll have taken the first step over—I'll see you on the other side!

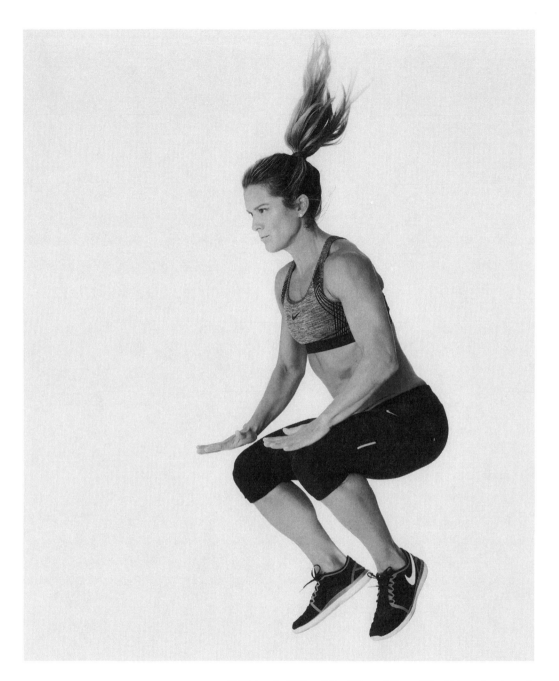

THE PROGRAM

2

Mind (AKA Breathe!)

Are you wondering why I begin by first focusing on the mind? It's not because most people always put the three in that specific order—mind, body, and spirit. It's first because lifting your mind should always be the first priority of your day. In fact, I'll be asking you to lift your mind right before and even during your workouts.

Here's why: your mind sets the stage. There are plenty of people who have great bodies who are unhappy, and there are plenty of people who have a clear mind who feel trapped in their own skin. Either of those situations always leads to a spirit that cannot fly as high as it could.

The entire premise of LIFTED is that you cannot separate the three, and the mind is the key to making lasting change to your body and spirit.

From my personal experience, going through so many highs and lows from the time I was a kid, one important thing that I discovered early—and what I want you to remember—is that you become your thoughts. That's because the thoughts and ideas we repeat in our minds eventually become what we believe about ourselves. What we believe about ourselves leads to the way we act and the actions we take as a result. Those actions eventually lead to habits, and what makes up the balance of our life is basically the habits we're tied to.

After all, we are creatures of habit.

When you finally realize how your thoughts are ultimately the foundation of your life, you'll suddenly see why you need to make sure your thoughts are on your side. I mean, think about it: if you constantly think you are fat or if you never stop telling yourself that you're not good enough, you don't just start believing that—you become that.

But what meditation does, among so many other things, is give you the chance to peek inside your head. It's a powerful tool that acts like a magnifying glass that lets you observe the thoughts going back and forth inside your head. But more importantly, it helps you recognize the thoughts that may be keeping you from being who you want to be—and making you who you are right now. It also allows you to understand that you have the power to let them go. They can be as inconsequential as a car driving past you on the street.

Maybe you just want to jump right into the Body portion and start breaking a sweat—and I'm with you. But maybe there's a lot happening behind the scenes in your mind right now that might make those workouts less productive. Maybe you think you're not good enough, or you don't believe you'll ever have the body you want because your parents are heavy, or you don't believe you're coordinated enough to exercise.

That's why I need you to start thinking about your mind like it's one big chemistry lab where you create every single day of your life by choosing what components to add to it. You are the alchemist, and it all starts with having the perfect environment to grow perfect thoughts—perfect thoughts that will eventually lead to perfect actions, then perfect habits, and, ultimately, the perfect life. (Okay, life will never be perfect, and neither will your thoughts, but your approach to life can be!)

YOUR MIND NEEDS A BREAK NOW AND THEN: We all know what it's like to have a million thoughts banging off the walls of our minds. Or more specifically, the same twenty thoughts going back and forth like a ping-pong match. For me it might go something like this:

Oh damn! I have to remember to pick up my laundry before five tonight.
I still can't believe Leslie said what she said about me last night. I'm so pissed!
I can't wait for vacation next week—is it Friday yet?
Hmm, I need to pick a restaurant for my birthday dinner . . . ugh! Can't decide!
ARGH! I have to pay my AMEX bill! Oh yeah, I'm gonna wait and do that next week.
Repeat.
Repeat.
Repeat.
And yes, unfortunately . . . repeat!!

If you had a computer running twenty programs over and over again—all at the same time—its system would quickly begin to overload, start running slower, and eventually freeze and shut down completely. It's the same thing with your brain and, ultimately, your body. You get worn out from thinking the same thoughts or, should I say, running the same programs—all day long.

I believe we have no idea how crazy our minds are most of the time and how distracted we are. Sometimes you don't even realize that all these thoughts are running in the background. But eventually, whether you're aware of them or not, all those thoughts lead to mental fatigue that, if left out of control, eventually translates into physical fatigue, keeping both your body and spirit from ever having a chance to fly higher.

I'll be the first to admit that I can be the biggest drama queen on the planet. I know, I know—you never would have guessed that, right? Some of my closest friends are probably reading this book right now and nodding their heads saying, "Oh yeah, she is!" But guess what? Most of my drama never actually happens. It's usually nothing more than something I've made up in my head!

Whenever our thoughts go wild—thoughts about the things we need to do, the things we haven't done yet, the things happening to those around us, and the things happening to ourselves—they overwhelm our mind . . . if we allow them to.

Sometimes these storylines about ourselves, our friends, our family, our coworkers—even our enemies or people we don't even know—aren't actually happening at all or don't even matter. Yet it's all those thoughts going around and around in your head that tether you and hold you back. The fact is that these thoughts will always come because most of us have a lot going on in our lives. But we don't need to be held captive to the ones that make no sense running in our background.

Meditation helps you get these thoughts under control. Just like you can train your muscles to perform at a higher level, meditation helps you train your mind to work in a more efficient way. It lets you practice processing thoughts every day so your mind knows how to deal with whatever thoughts may try to hijack it.

The more you continue to meditate, the easier it will be to let certain thoughts come and go and to ignore any storylines you shouldn't be following in the first place. But for now all I'm asking you to do is try to start sweeping out these thoughts with ten minutes of meditation a day. Ten minutes to make space in your brain so you can be happier, more productive, and start living in the *now*.

What You'll Find When You LIFT Your Mind: The Benefits of Meditation

When it comes to all the benefits meditation offers, I'll be honest: everyone is different. With all the benefits of meditation just coming to the forefront of conversations right now, I bet there are more waiting to be discovered. But from what we *do* know, it's almost unbelievable what physiological effects you may expect to see from just simply crossing your legs, breathing, and focusing.

If you thought meditation was only about reducing stress, here are just a few of the things that may be happening behind the scenes as you become more aware of your thoughts and lift your mind even higher than ever.

Meditation Fortifies Your Immune System

Meditation has an amazing ability to increase your feeling of control and decrease your negative emotions simultaneously. Not only does that make you feel better, but according to research, reducing your chronic psychological stress may improve the longevity of immune cells.[1] Fewer sick days? Sign me up!

Meditation Builds a Better Body

Later in this chapter I'll show you how and when to meditate, but know that you'll be meditating before and during your exercise routine. Why? Most people are in such a rush that they jump right into their workouts. But if you don't give yourself a moment to free your mind through meditation, to take a certain amount of time to get in touch with yourself, it's possible to get less from your workouts and be more prone to injury because you're less focused. You may have other things on your mind that are distracting you and keeping you from using proper form or putting in as much effort.

Take this from a former pro athlete. The time I spent before games was sacred. I *knew* that without it, I would not perform at the level I was capable of. That's the reason many top athletes use meditation. They know that in order to perform better and be more focused on their training, they need to focus on their mind before their muscles. That's what gives LIFTED an edge over most workout programs: you'll be getting a taste of what the best of the best use to make them healthier and stronger. And if it works for them, I can promise you: it will work for you.

Meditation Lets You Sleep More Soundly

It's almost funny how some people think that meditation is nothing but taking a nap with your legs crossed—the key to meditation is to relax but stay awake so you can be aware of your thoughts. But as it turns out, there's a lot of evidence that suggests that regular meditation helps lower levels of both physical and mental arousal, which can improve your sleep time and lower your risk of insomnia.[2] There is even evidence that spending longer periods meditating may decrease your need for sleep![3] So if you start noticing that you're sleeping less but feeling even more refreshed every morning than usual, chances are you have meditation to thank for that.

True story: I used to get so mad at my ex-girlfriend when I told her how tired I was, and she would suggest I meditate. What I wanted was a nap! The fact is that we don't always have time for a nap. Yet just a few minutes of meditation can stir up some real energy.

Meditation Boosts Your Brain

Meditation doesn't just help you connect and disconnect with your thoughts; it just might make the brain they're in a lot stronger. Studies have shown that regular meditation may make the white matter of your brain more efficient at improving self-regulation—and reducing and possibly preventing mental disorders—by helping to increase myelin, the fatty substance that surrounds nerve cells.[4]

Regular meditation has also been shown to improve blood flow to the brain, improve cognitive function, and may even prevent the atrophy of gray matter that happens as we age.[5] In fact, research has shown that meditating for as little as one month can significantly raise your IQ by reducing the changes in cognitive function and intelligence that occur due to stress.[6] To put it simply: the more you meditate, the less stress you'll have holding your brain back.

Meditation Reduces Your Aches and Pains

Even just practicing meditation for a short period of time has been shown to reduce the expression of genes that produce inflammatory responses in stress-related pathways.[7] What exactly does that mean? It means that devoting just a few minutes a day to meditation may reduce the harmful, chronic forms of inflammation that ultimately cause the degeneration of tissue that can lead to disease. Taking time to meditate has also been shown to significantly improve a person's ability to manage chronic pain, so by taking a pause every day, you're helping to prevent pain from ever standing in your way from lifting off.[8]

Meditation Reduces Your Wrong Reactions

It's a pretty simple concept that if we focus on what we're doing, we're probably going to do it better. Yet most times when we're reactive, we're reacting to an emotion. So when we're not in control of our thoughts, we're reacting to an emotion and just going for it. But when we can watch that thought arise and realize that we're having an emotional reaction to something and that we're about to react in a way that isn't really who we are or what we're all about, we can detach from it and make better decisions at that moment.

In other words, meditation teaches you how to put a little space between yourself and certain reactions led by emotion. Over time you'll find yourself reacting to emotions in a different way. You'll begin counting to ten and discover that you can take the time to breathe and create more space between yourself and whatever crazy, irrational, toxic reaction you were about to have. It gives you that time to reflect on how you may react to certain situations that may happen during your day, so you always put your best foot forward. Remember when your granny or your mom told you to count to ten to cool off and take a few deep breaths? That old adage rings true!

Meditation Smartens Your Decisions

How many times have you grabbed a piece of chocolate just because you read a stressful email? Or found yourself looking in the fridge for the twentieth time when you have a big project due the next day? It's because you're letting yourself be led around on a leash by your thoughts. The thoughts are entering your head, but instead of addressing them, you end up unconsciously finding something to distract yourself. And for many people that distraction can easily be food.

I've been there. But when I meditate I become more instantly aware of certain thoughts and the things that are really pressing on my mind. It allow me to say, "There's that thought again for the tenth time!" And every time I do that—every time I acknowledge that thought—I've most likely just stopped myself ten times from going into my kitchen and opening the refrigerator door. It allows me to manage as an observer the stressful thoughts that come into my head, just like I do when I'm meditating—but now I'm able to do it in my waking daily life. I'm no longer run by my thoughts—I'm running my life. I'm awake!

You'll start becoming aware of the thoughts that are driving you to make decisions that aren't good for you too, but don't just take my word for it. Research has shown that using mindfulness-based meditation effectively decreases binge eating and emotional eating in people who typically engage in that type of behavior.[9] Whether it's because meditation decreases stress, depression, and anxiety—three major reasons why most of us find ourselves turning to food as an answer—isn't exactly known yet. But having all three decrease just by spending a few minutes meditating makes it worth trying, doesn't it?

Meditation Lowers Your Blood Pressure

In the next chapter you're going to experience the workout portion of LIFTED that will burn fat, build muscle, and boost your metabolism. These routines will also improve your cardiovascular fitness and help lower your blood pressure, but that's not the only part of this program that can affect your heart. Meditation has just as much to offer.

Regular meditation has been shown to improve everything from your resting heart rate, mean arterial blood pressure, and even your systolic and diastolic blood pressure.[10] Just think about that. It's really the lowest hanging fruit possible when you look at it: you can lower your blood pressure and live a healthier life just by taking the time to breathe. The simple act of focusing on your breath and spending a few minutes with your thoughts creates such an amazing physiological benefit such as lowering your blood pressure. Can you imagine if instead of instantly going to meds, meditation was considered a first stop to curing some of the most common diseases like high blood pressure? I mean, sign me up!

Before You Start . . .
Don't Let Time Talk You Out of It

If you say you don't have time to meditate, then stop yourself right there. The next time you say "I don't have time for [blank]," I want you to then repeat that phrase using these words instead: "It's not important enough for me to [blank]."

Isn't it funny that we often always seem to find time for the things we want to do, yet never seem to have time for the things we may be less excited to do? In fact, I'm willing to bet that on any given day you can find at least one moment—if not many moments—when, if you're *truly honest* with yourself, you'll admit that you're probably wasting time.

I understand. No one likes to admit they're spending their time unwisely because it can make us seem as if we're lazy. But the fact is that we all waste time to some extent. If you add up how many minutes a day you check your phone, go to your social media sites, watch television, or surf the Internet, you'll be surprised just how much time you really have that you thought didn't exist. So before you say you don't have time to meditate, I want you to do this:

LOOK FOR THE TIME EATERS. If you're like a lot of people I've worked with who didn't think they had time to meditate, the easiest place to find wasted minutes will probably be how much time you spend on social media. But I can't assume where you may have more time to meditate. All I know is that those pockets of wasted time are always there to be found. And if you're not finding them, it may be a question of not being honest with yourself.

If you suspect that you might talk yourself out of meditating because you have no time, then before you start the LIFTED program I want you to do a time audit of yourself over the next few days. From the moment you wake up until the moment you go to bed, I want you to write down how you're spending all the minutes of your day.

And be honest with the numbers, because if anyone is going to know you're lying, it's going to be yourself.

Once you have that time audit finished, just keep it handy as you start LIFTED. If at any time, you ever feel you don't have a few minutes to spare to meditate, I want you to immediately reflect back on that sheet of paper and look at all the things you choose to spend time on instead. Now that you're aware of all the health benefits that meditation can bring, I can pretty much say with absolute certainty that you won't find much on that list worth more to your mind, body, and spirit than the few minutes I'm asking for from you each day.

LOOK FOR IDLE TIME. As you get more comfortable with meditation, you'll find that you can do it in places you would never expect. I've had clients able to do it on the subway, on plane flights, and even sitting and waiting for their child at baseball practice or dance class.

Again, I would never expect you to be able to do this if you're new to meditation. Just opening your eyes and noticing that others are looking at you might be a little unsettling. But know that what sounds unbelievable now will come—so get excited about it!

In the meantime I want you to keep an eye out for those little moments in your life when you might find yourself waiting. Because sometimes it's not always our fault for wasting time—it's life that's the culprit. Whether it's sitting in a coffeehouse waiting for your order, standing in line at the post office, or being the first one at the board meeting, there are plenty of moments every day when we wish time would move faster and, sadly, usually reach for our phones. Soon, instead of entertaining yourself, you'll know how to LIFT yourself during those moments when you're made to wait.

Expect to have more time. Sometimes the more Type A you are, the more likely you might feel that meditation is a waste of your time. After all, you could be getting something done in that time when you feel like you're doing absolutely nothing. But one unexpected benefit of meditating is that, by investing just a few minutes each day, you might actually free up even more time in your day as a result.

It works like this: Because daily meditation makes it much easier to stay relaxed and more focused, many people quickly discover that they're able to concentrate better and work more effectively throughout the day. It also makes you more energized, so many people find that they end up doing certain jobs and tasks even faster, leaving them more free time afterward to do the things they'd rather do. So the time you put in meditating is time you'll most likely get back—plus a few minutes of free time at the least. It's a time trade-off that's hard to turn down!

LIFT Yourself:
Put Your Headphones On and Enjoy the Silence

I often sit with my headphones in my ears—but I'm not listening to any music. I'll just close my eyes and meditate. People assume I'm listening to music so they leave me alone, and I feel less distracted and vulnerable.

Ready To LIFT Your Mind? Here's How

Meditation

Meditation can come in a lot of different forms. As an athlete, I experienced it for the first time in a much different way from how I'm about to show you. At first it didn't come in the purest sense of crossing my legs, putting my hands on my knees, and focusing on my breath as it does for me today. But when I was younger, before every game I would take myself to a quiet place and disconnect from the rest of my day.

No matter what else was happening in my life at that time, whether I had a test coming up or was dealing with a relationship problem, I would step back from it all and make my game the most important thing of my life. I would take that time to focus on the now, and through that focus the game always became the most important thing in that moment. I didn't realize what I was doing back then, but now I see that I was putting myself in a very meditative state of mind. That focus became more and more important to me as I went from being a kid into making basketball my career.

What I discovered as an athlete and what others noticed about me was that when I performed at my absolute best on the court, there was always such a calmness about me. My coaches always used to comment on how I always seemed to have so much poise, even when I was playing at my hardest. I could be sprinting full-out down the court, but if you looked at me, I was so controlled. My face was never frenzied—instead, I looked free.

Today I meditate the exact way I'm about to show you, but the feeling I get afterward is the same feeling I had when I was on the court. It's the same powerful and harmonious energy I've felt in other moments of my life, from letting go on the dance floor, catching waves in Montauk or Costa Rica, or just running on the West Side Highway. Moments that felt effortless because I was simply *being*—I was simply *doing*.

Meditation can be anything that calms you down, gets you in the moment, and keeps you in the moment. But for now, when I ask you to LIFT your mind, here is exactly what I'd like you to do:

Set a Distraction-less Stage

Find the time that's best for your mind. I think trial and error is the best way to handle anything in life. I would never be bold enough to tell you what will work best for you—all I'll ever do is give you some of the tools. So which time is best to meditate is up to you—and that time may change from day to day. There will always be people who are best in the evening or find themselves more focused in the afternoons.

That just doesn't happen to be me.

I personally like to do it in the morning because, just like my workouts, I feel like it sets the pace for the rest of my day, and there's a lot of benefit to having the rest of your day being a little calmer. When you do it right, the peace of mind you'll experience is a feeling you can then carry into the rest of your morning, afternoon, and evening—so why not start fresh? Besides, in addition to that, it makes you less likely to skip it. The more we wait to do things in the day, the more susceptible we become to blowing them off.

Another reason why mornings often work best for many people is that you're usually dressed for the occasion—or, should I say, not as dressed. When you meditate, it's always smarter to avoid any restrictive clothing that may distract you from being in the moment. Mind you—once you become practiced at being able to meditate any place, what you're wearing most likely won't ever be of any concern. But when you're just starting out, dressing in clothing that makes you feel more relaxed and less restricted can help you make the most of your meditation time and give yourself your best attention possible. So try to stick with mornings, when I doubt you're dressed in anything but what makes you the most relaxed.

Give Yourself at Least Ten Minutes of Time

The one thing I'll never tell you to do is meditate for only a certain number of minutes. Once you begin to LIFT your mind, if your life allows it, you have my complete permission to meditate for as long as you want each day. The longer you do, the more you'll feel purified, refreshed, and good to go. What you'll begin to find is that there are layers you can get through with more time. The deeper the water, the more peaceful. It just takes time to shed layers and dive deeper.

Are there a lot of practices of meditation that recommend meditating for a minimum of twenty minutes in the morning and twenty minutes at night? Absolutely, and I get how meditating that much will improve your life—I've actually tried it. I just think that for most people, it's very hard to find that much time in the day. So even if you're not pressed for time, a great place to start is simply by devoting a minimum of ten minutes a day.

If you can't imagine meditating for longer than fifteen minutes, you may surprise yourself sooner than you think. That's because the more often you meditate, the more you'll find yourself able to meditate for longer periods of time. Not just because it will become easier to get yourself in that moment, but also because you'll begin to see the value of meditation and want to do it more.

Finally, if ten minutes still feels like a lot of time, let me just say this to you: I believe there is something sacred and special about sitting down with yourself. I want you to remember that this time is about showing yourself some respect. I want you to think about these ten minutes of meditation almost as if you're bowing down to yourself. So before you decide how many minutes you're going to meditate, ask yourself how many minutes you deserve to give yourself. I think you'll find you may raise that number a little higher because deep down, you know you're worth it.

Let Someone Else Watch the Clock

I always set a timer because it's just human nature to need to know. Inevitably—and I've seen it not just with clients but with myself—you're going to be into minute seven and find yourself thinking, "Oh my God, it's been so long!" and opening your eyes to check in with a clock to see what time it is or how much longer you have to go.

That's entirely normal, which is why I want meditation to be as palatable and natural of a process as possible. Instead, set a timer so you'll have the peace of mind of knowing you won't accidentally lose yourself in the moment and spend more time than you may have. Just be sure to tack on an extra minute or two at the beginning to give yourself time to settle into your session. Then, if possible, choose an alarm that's soft and soothing instead of loud and obnoxious so that you come out of every session more relaxed and at peace.

Choose Your Safe Spot to Succeed

If you're new to meditation, the whole process can leave you feeling a little bit vulnerable—and that's understandable. It's entirely natural to feel that way whenever you try anything for the first time in your life. But trust me when I tell you that won't be the case in just a few months' time. You'll soon be surprised at the many places you'll find yourself stealing away moments to meditate in places you would never expect to. But for now I want you to look for a place where you can be entirely by yourself—a place that makes you feel safe and at peace.

It's important to set yourself up for success, which is why I'm a big believer in carving out a quiet, comfortable place where you can allow yourself to fully experience meditation without wondering what people are thinking about you. A place where you don't have to worry about your dog coming in and licking your face or your kids running past you and tugging at your shirt. Eventually you'll surprise yourself at being able to meditate almost anywhere, but for now I discovered that many of my clients find using their bedroom is a great starting point. Just make sure there is no clutter lying around, which can sometimes cause a distraction.

Allow Your Body to Find Its Preferred Posture

Everybody has this image of how to sit during meditation. You know the one: with legs crossed and your forearms resting on your thighs, hands folded. Personally I love this position because it makes me feel like I'm part of the ancient tradition of meditation. Just sitting in this position really feels like it's allowing my body language to say, "I'm open to this moment." So if you're up for it, that would be the posture to start with.

But I also get that we all have different mindsets, so if that posture makes you feel silly, then I don't want you to stick with it. We also all have different bodies of all different shapes and sizes. So even if you're up to use it, if this pose is a position that makes you feel awkward, even in the slightest, then the same rules apply. I would rather have you in a position that's not distracting, so just sit down and position yourself in whatever way feels best for your body, puts your mind at ease, and makes your spirit soar.

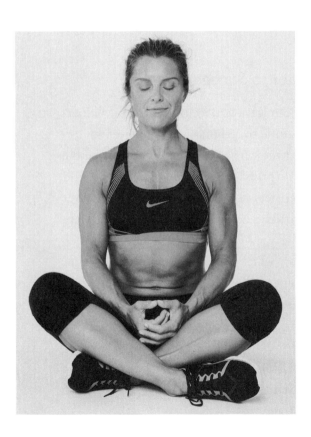

If you prefer sitting up against your sofa so you have more support for your back, that's fine. If you would rather sit on a chair with your feet on the ground because that's more comfortable for you, that works too. You have my full permission to run through a bunch of options so you can weed out what may distract you. So take the time beforehand to test drive some positions or seating arrangements to see which one feels best for your body. If any distract you from being in the moment, then don't feel compelled to stay in them *just* because you think that's how everyone else does it.

However, I don't want you to be *too* comfortable. Whatever posture you choose, you should be sitting upright—not lying down, which isn't the best because it usually induces sleep, as opposed to sitting upright, which lets you remain in a state of awareness. So avoid lying down at all costs because I need you to be stimulated and aware to facilitate the flow of energy.

Finally, if you do choose to sit in a chair, just make sure you grab one with a flat seat that doesn't make it easy to tilt it back. Your feet should also rest comfortably on the floor. So if your feet dangle, place a box or something stable on the floor that you can place your feet on.

Get in Tune from Top to Bottom

Be somewhat aware of your air. When you sit down and actually make yourself aware of your breath, it's a little bit like being near the ocean. You can hear the waves going out and coming back in. There is just something about the ocean and how big and endless it is that's comforting because it can remind you of how small our stresses are compared to its vastness.

Some people assume they need to measure their breath as they meditate, counting how many seconds they inhale and how many seconds they exhale. Or others think they should always breathe through the belly and never the chest. The problem, I feel, is that all that instruction on how to do something that we do naturally every single second suddenly makes it no longer natural.

Your breathing shouldn't be turned into some regimented ritual you need to monitor as you meditate. If you do that too much, you'll never spend enough time getting the most from the moment. However, there are a few things I do that I find incredibly helpful.

Let your breath flow where it wants to: just breathe as your body wants to breathe at that moment, then make yourself aware of how you're breathing. I don't want you to try to change the way you're breathing or wonder whether you're breathing through your chest or your belly. And don't count how many seconds you're inhaling versus how many seconds you're exhaling; instead, as you meditate, try to simply *notice* your breath to see what it's doing and where it's going rather than try to change it.

Some days when I feel stressed out I'll notice that my heart rate is elevated and my breath is much shorter and centered more in my chest. Other times when I meditate in the evening after I've spent some time relaxing at the beach, I'll notice that my breath is much deeper, flows at a much slower pace, and always fills my belly. You'll likely find the same nuances.

Meditation is probably one of the only times in your day when you observe your breathing and really tune into how your body is reacting to the things happening around it. By being observant of your breathing, you can see that both stressful moments and peaceful moments make your body react in certain ways that you may not be acknowledging.

Through the nose is a yes. I find that breathing through my nose calms me down and helps me focus on my breath. But beyond that, research has shown that nasal breathing is always better because of what your nose was designed to do in the first place: filter out bad particles, kill viruses and bacteria, and warm the air before it reaches your lungs. Breathing through your nose also allows a greater amount of oxygen to be taken in with each breath. The more oxygen your body can extract, the more energized you'll feel after you meditate.

Breathe for a few—then close the two. When I first begin any meditation session, I also like my eyes to be open for the first few breaths. It allows me to observe my surroundings and places me in that moment, so when I finally do close my eyes, I can let go of any distractions that may come as I begin. For some reason, knowing what's around me makes any distractions that might come my way less distracting.

Let the Sounds Come to You

Even though I would prefer you try to find a nice quiet spot to start, there will always be noises in the background for most of us—and that's entirely fine. I remember the first few times I began meditating in my apartment there was actually a jackhammer pounding away outside. What was my immediate reaction? I told myself that I couldn't meditate. But in all honesty, what I didn't realize at the time was how that noisy jackhammer was just part of my meditation experience.

That's why I don't want you to try to block whatever remaining sounds you hear as you meditate but rather bring them into your experience. Try making yourself aware of the sounds closest to you as you meditate, then begin to make yourself aware of the sounds that are further and further away from you.

Trust me! Doing this simple trick keeps you in the moment because it prevents you from thinking about yesterday or tomorrow. By being aware of the noises within your orbit, you will keep yourself grounded to the present.

Scan Your Skin—Then Go Within

When you're not in tune with your body, you don't listen to the messages it's trying to send you. Meditation can make you more aware of little aches and pains that can't seem to get your attention or which parts of your body may need a little more love.

Start small by just letting yourself become aware of the parts of yourself that are touching other parts. For example, how the skin of your hands feels on your thighs, how your legs feel crossed over each other, or how your hair feels along the back of your neck or on your shoulders. From there work your way along your body, and try to make yourself aware of every part.

You might compare how one arm feels compared to the other arm. You may decide to listen to every finger and every toe, every joint and every point of skin. Your body may not have anything to tell you at all at that moment, but just taking time to listen to any complaints will make your body more appreciative.

As You Begin Your Ascent...

Turn your mind into an open sky. One of the biggest misconceptions about meditation that people have is that they think they need to stop, well, *thinking*!

It's the main reason why people often believe they can't meditate in the first place. The first time they try, they realize that they're thinking too much and assume there's some trick to it—one they can never master—so they immediately give up. But you can't stop thinking because that's impossible, and you can't stop thoughts from popping into your mind. Once you realize that *not thinking* isn't the objective, you'll feel a lot less pressure. Phew!

Instead, picture yourself sitting on a ledge, looking down at yourself and watching your thoughts go by like moving cars or people. Or imagine yourself lying down on the ground, picture your mind like the sky, and let your thoughts be clouds. I love this analogy because clouds come in all shapes and sizes, just as there are many kinds of thoughts that run both big and small. Sometimes your thoughts might be darker, larger, and intense. Other days your thoughts might be light and fluffy. And every time you sit down to meditate, it's going to be a different sky.

But the main reason I love having clients think of their thoughts as clouds is that it's important to simply observe your thoughts just coming and going. You need to watch your thoughts from a distance and recognize them as just things that come and go—things that eventually pass you by.

The point is, don't worry that they are there. The presence of your thoughts is entirely normal, and now, through meditation, they are being recognized and removed, one by one. So if you think your mind seems quiet now, try meditating a few days in a row—you'll be surprised when you notice a newfound mental peace.

Final note: don't be surprised if certain thoughts you *think* you've never thought about suddenly seem to come out of left field. These are thoughts that have always been present in your mind. It's just that with so many thoughts screaming for attention inside your head, these may be thoughts that try their best to get noticed but are never heard over the shouting.

Place Space Between Your Thoughts

As you meditate, you will find your mind attach to a thought because that's what it does. It's habitual, and we *are* human beings after all! But the second you notice that you're attached to a thought, here's what I want you to do:

First, calmly label that moment for what it is: *thinking*. And then bring yourself back to your breath and back to that present rhythmic place.

Then try—really hard—not to be upset or disappointed in yourself. It's easy to get very frustrated (trust me, I've seen it—and felt it—a gazillion times). So when it first happens to you—and it will every single time you meditate—don't say to yourself, "There I go! I'm thinking again. I can't be here! I can't do this!"

The thing is, you're doing it. Even when that happens, you're still meditating the right way. In fact, you could be meditating for twenty-five years, and you'll never sit down and not have a thought. So getting mad at yourself not only doesn't help anything but is pointless because what's happening is entirely natural.

Your first time through, you may find yourself attached to a thought every few seconds. But I promise you that as you continue to meditate, what you'll see is that the space between your thoughts will start to open up a little bit more. That's really all you can hope for—more space between each thought.

It's Not About Planning—It's About Purging

Meditation isn't the time to think about solving anything that's happening in your life, especially the thoughts you're sitting back and observing.

I want you to simply sit and observe your mind's inner dialogue. What are you thinking? What are you feeling? Let your mind continue to think, but don't engage in any way. For example, if you suddenly think, "I have to do laundry tonight," do your best not to react to the thought. Rather than getting annoyed by the fact that you have to do it or start to think about what you need to throw in the washer, recognize that you are having a thought that you have to do laundry, then let that thought float on by.

I think a lot of Type A people like myself tend to believe that if we spend more time thinking about a problem, we can work it out a lot faster. So when meditation starts making us aware of certain problems we need to face, we sometimes have a tendency to get excited about those things and want to immediately focus on them during meditation in order to solve them. I've actually jumped out of meditation to do something and then stopped myself. Talk about a powerful habit!

But like I said, meditation is all about finding value in creating space between those thoughts versus working through them all. I want you to remember that you have the rest of the day to deal with the rest of your day. So give yourself those ten minutes, and as thoughts pop into your head, don't try to solve them—just let them slowly fade away.

As You Return to Reality, End Your Session Slowly

Once your time is up, don't just jump right up and get back into life. Start off by making yourself aware of the physical reality around you for at least fifteen to thirty seconds. Then, very slowly, open your eyes and get attuned to your surroundings, but don't get up just yet. Instead, remain perfectly still in your meditative spot and sit in that moment. Soak in that feeling because that's a magical moment when you have the most clarity, the most peace, and the most space between your thoughts.

Give Yourself Credit for Anything—And Even Nothing

Who cares if you had a lot of stress and couldn't dismiss that while you were meditating? Is it your fault that one day your life was so stressful that you couldn't keep yourself from being distracted? Know that there are always different types of days, so no matter what, if you sat down to meditate, that is accomplishment. That's how I see it—and so should you!

First of all, having stress is totally normal. A lot of people are always going to have something that's weighing on their minds, whether that's work, family, relationships, or any number of situations that can cause worry. But I don't want there ever to be a day when you walk away thinking you didn't do a good job meditating. All that should ever matter to you is that you took time out of your day for yourself.

That alone should leave you feeling fulfilled. And if anything, know you'll have days when you'll feel fantastic, and you'll have days that are not so fantastic. But I can guarantee you that just by sitting there, you started to create a little bit of space between your thoughts, even if you think you didn't. And that's what it's about.

Solo or Social—You Decide!

If you're new to meditation, the very thought of trying to place space between your thoughts while someone else is in the room might seem nuts. But that doesn't mean it's not doable. If you have a friend trying LIFTED at the same time or someone you know who meditates on a daily basis, you're more than welcome to meditate with a friend to add a social component to it.

Personally I believe the spirit works in such crazy ways, and I can honestly say there is a different type of energy when like-minded people come together. I've gone to guided meditation sessions where there is an energy in the room that I felt not only individually but also collectively. It's the same energy I try to bring into every class I teach. So once you get the hang of it and feel comfortable meditating by yourself, give it a try with a partner or a group. I promise that what you'll experience will not only be as effective as doing it alone but will also bring an entirely different type of tranquility to your sessions.

3

Body (AKA Sweat!)

I'm not most trainers. But then again, I'm not looking to train you so that you look great for summer, are ready for some upcoming wedding, or fit better in a pair of jeans.

Instead, my goal with LIFTED is to train you for life.

You wake up every day in this skin—it's here to stay. So you need to make a commitment to having the best body you can in this life. It's not about vanity—it's about happiness. I've always believed that people can make their own happiness in a lot of ways. But when you feel comfortable in your skin and begin to experience how wonderful you feel when your body is as healthy as it can be, that's such a fantastic place to start from.

When you're less in tune with your body, you suddenly find yourself more powerless and less in control of so many other—if not all—facets of your life. If you don't take care of it, your body may prevent you from being able to experience many joyful activities in life or having the confidence to even try, both of which can also keep your mind and spirit down as well.

Have you ever wanted to not go out because you didn't feel comfortable in your clothes? Have you ever lacked the energy to do something fun or couldn't discover the confidence within yourself to give it a shot because you were nervous that being out of shape would cause you to fail? It's in those instances, which may happen more often than you might want to admit, when your perception of your body keeps you from lifting yourself up and prevents that continual state of growth.

This workout is not just about calories burned, building lean muscle, or cardiovascular health—those are all just bonuses. These workouts are the foundation of the rest of your life.

Your commitment to your body is ultimately a commitment to your overall success and happiness.

Making a commitment to your body eliminates the need for negotiation. It's about realizing that you're never choosing between your career or your health, or your family or your health. It's about realizing that to achieve ultimate success in all parts of your life, you need to take care of the vehicle that's taking you through that life.

If you're ready to make that commitment to your body, here's how LIFTED will help you make the most of that promise.

A Great Workout
Never Neglects Your Body

When it comes to fitness, the question most people ask is this: How can I put the least amount of effort in yet get the most results? For the longest time the fitness industry was built around the promise of big results from little effort. But that's not how you should ever look at exercise. If that's always been your game plan, it's probably why what you've been doing to reshape your body has never been as productive as you had always hoped.

For most people the main reason they never see great results is because they honestly never put in enough time to get great results. It takes being committed to *move* your body through some form of exercise for a minimum of thirty minutes a day, five to six days a week, which is exactly what you'll be doing throughout the four-week LIFTED program.

I know that might be mind-blowing and seem unrealistic, and if you've already thrown your hands up at that statement, I get it. If you're new to exercise, I'm sure you were hoping for something along the lines of two to three times per week like most trainers would suggest.

But I promise you: not every day will be extreme, and I want you to look at this from a 360-degree perspective. Even though this is the physical part of the program, the upside to this isn't just rooted in the physical; you're doing this because it's going to set the pace for the rest of your day. You will experience ancillary benefits that reach far beyond just the calories you'll be burning or the muscles you'll be working. That said . . .

A Great Workout
Never Destroys Your Body

Being a trainer in New York City, I see this pervasive mentality that if a workout doesn't leave you throwing up in a corner or feeling completely annihilated, there is no value in it. Well, know this: that's just not the case.

The fitness industry has shifted from "do as little as possible" to too far in the opposite direction. I see trainers with the hashtag #nodaysoff all over their Instagram and Twitter accounts. And don't get me wrong—I remember those days too. I remember that point in my life when I felt the exact same thing. But it took me thirty-five years to understand the value of maximizing your time when you exercise as well as the importance of rest.

I'm Type A—okay, maybe triple A—so I get that desire to push yourself as far as you possibly can. But a workout should not only break your body down but give it enough time to build itself back up into something even better. Push it too hard—or keep it from getting enough time to rest—and all your hard work won't just lead to fewer results; it will set your body down the path of getting injured and thrown out of the game entirely.

The LIFTED Advantage

My approach to fitness is simple. The Body portion of the four-week LIFTED program involves a weekly commitment to a six-days-on, one-day-off exercise routine that breaks down like this:

- Day One: Work your upper body.
- Day Two: Work your lower body.
- Day Three: Work your abs.
- Day Four: Do thirty minutes of cardio (high-intensity interval training).
- Day Five: Work your upper body with a more intense program.
- Day Six: Work your lower body with a more intense program.
- Day Seven: Rest.

Each day you work out you'll perform a three-and-a-half-minute dynamic warmup routine to get your blood flowing and your body ready to exercise. After you finish your workout, you'll then perform a series of stretches that take only a few minutes as well—and you're done. Your basic version of the workout is finished in less than forty minutes!

As for the exercises in the program, I've always been a huge advocate of quality over quantity. You don't have to spend hours exercising to reach your goals; when it comes to strength training, most people work their muscles longer and harder than they need to. Not only is that not the best way to achieve faster results, but it also increases your risk of overtraining and injuring yourself. Instead, my program relies on a variety of tried and true, common-sense techniques.

1. **You'll burn more fat *as* you exercise.** The more muscles you can work at once, the more calories your body has to burn, which is why my workout plan keeps your entire body constantly challenged and engaged. My program uses a variety of multijoint moves that train several muscles to work together instead of isolating just one, giving you the best full-body workout in less time. Honestly, this is the kind of workout you can squeeze in at lunchtime if you need to.

   More importantly, they're arranged in a way that melts more fat as you build muscle. This is where high-intensity interval training (HIIT) comes in—a training technique in which you give all-out, one hundred percent effort within quick, intense bursts of exercise, followed by short, sometimes active, recovery periods. This type of training spikes your heart rate and ultimately burns more fat in less time and, in my opinion, offers the best bang for your buck.

2. **You'll burn more fat *after* you exercise.** The multimuscle exercises and HIIT-style workouts you'll be using not only burn plenty of calories *as* you do them, but they also help create an oxygen deficit in your body from the all-out effort they require. The more oxygen you use during your workout, the harder your body has to work afterward to restore itself to a level of homeostasis (a fancy word for when your body returns to a normal state of balance).

This is where the real magic begins. This effect—known as excess post-oxygen consumption, or EPOC—results in your body using more oxygen to fill its energy stores as well as to bring your body temperature, heart rate, and hormone and oxygen levels back to normal. All that extra effort takes energy, which is why your body burns calories at a higher overall rate long after you exercise.

The effect—otherwise known as the *afterburn effect*—can last for a few minutes or up to twenty-four to forty-eight hours, depending on what type of exercises or routines you do. Fortunately for your body, because of the routines in LIFTED, you can count on your afterburn effect lasting at least twenty-four to forty-eight hours. Pretty amazing, right?

3. **You'll burn more calories when you're *not* exercising.** It works like this: the more lean muscle you have on your body, the higher your metabolism revs. Why? Because lean muscle tissue requires a certain amount of energy each day just to maintain and rebuild itself (about three times more calories than body fat!). The end result: increasing lean muscle tissue turns you into a fat-burning furnace night and day—even when you're just standing still or as you sleep. It takes the right full-body workout performed often enough to both preserve the muscle you already have and build even more lean muscle, which is precisely what this workout is all about.

But beyond all these calorie-burning benefits, what you can expect from using the workout portion of LIFTED goes far beyond fat loss. LIFTED helps you . . .

Connect Your Mind with Your Muscles

Beyond burning more calories, the program also leaves your muscles no choice but to be in better sync with each another. Many of the exercises in the program use a combination of compound moves that develop functional strength—that is, strength in your day-to-day life—that can help improve your performance and body awareness performing everyday activities. So as you burn fat and build muscle, you're also making more of a mind-body connection that will mean more speed, more power, and more balance when moving in any direction, whether on or off the field or just in life.

Bring Balance Back to Your Body

A lot of the daily aches and pains most people have aren't typically the result of something they did; it's about something they *didn't* do. Even if you work out regularly already, chances are you're muscularly imbalanced, due in part because you're focusing too much on the muscles you can see in the mirror and ignoring the muscles you can't. My LIFTED workout helps correct those flaws by training your body not just from top to bottom but also from front to back equally so you'll target every muscle group every week for a more complete physique.

Keep Your Body Guessing

Once your muscles get used to any exercise or workout routine, they, unfortunately, get smarter. Do the same routine over and over again, and your body begins to learn how to do that same routine more efficiently to conserve energy. The problem: once it adapts, your body burns less fat and calories from the same workout.

That's why a lot of people who stick with the same program start to see fewer results—and sometimes stop seeing results altogether (a condition referred to as *plateauing*). My program keeps your muscles from adapting by changing certain variables—the amount of repetitions you'll perform, the amount of time you'll do certain exercises, and how long you'll rest between circuits—every single week. That way you'll avoid plateauing and consistently challenge your body's limits so you boost your calorie-burning potential in *every* single workout.

LIFT at Your Level

Unlike a lot of exercise programs that are structured to be a one-size-fits-all program, my workout adapts to match your current fitness level. As you begin the plan you can either perform each exercise as described or make each one of them either easier or more challenging. Here's how it works:

- If you can't quite perform any exercise and need to float for now instead of lift, you'll find an option called "Until you're ready to fly!" at the end of each exercise description that will make the move possible.
- If you're already at an advanced fitness level and want to soar even more with an exercise, you'll also find an option called "Lift yourself higher!" This will show you how to turn up the volume on that particular exercise. That way, as you become fitter or feel the need to dial things back a bit, you can instantly make adjustments to the LIFTED program so you can continue to see results.

Dress for Success

To make the most of your workout, wearing the right clothes can make a world of difference. My suggestions?

Workout clothes: Your first choice should always be to wear light, breathable clothing that fits well and lets you move but isn't too loose and baggy. That way you'll be able to see the shape of your body during certain moves to check your form until you get the hang of them. Final suggestion: look for clothing that's either 100 percent cotton, a blended cotton mix, or a specially designed fabric like Dri-Fit. (You want clothing that will allow air to flow around your skin so sweat evaporates faster to keep you cool and comfortable.)

Sports bra: For the ladies, pick a sports bra with nonadjustable straps, extra support, and material that wicks away moisture for comfort.

Shoes: I personally prefer wearing a cross-training shoe over a running shoe. Some of the moves in the LIFTED workout require you to move laterally. A cross-trainer will give your ankles just enough support for any side-to-side movements as well as enough cushioning and traction to keep you from slipping while doing certain challenging exercises.

Fly for Free

No gym? No problem. Even though some of the more advanced versions of certain exercises in this program may require weights or medicine balls, the only equipment you'll ever need is something sturdy to lean on (to do a wall sit), a chair (to do dips), and an exercise mat (if you're doing any of the floor exercises on a hard surface and need a little comfort)—and that's it. So say goodbye to any excuses you might have had because you didn't have access to fitness equipment. You can do my routine in your living room, in a park, on vacation in your hotel room, or even on a balcony in said hotel room—the list of places you could put your body through its paces is endless.

The Basics

BEFORE YOU LIFT YOURSELF . . .
DO THE DYNAMIC WARMUP

The days of stretching before a workout are over! (But don't worry—I've saved a few stretches for the end of your workouts that I'll show you later.) Instead, you'll be warming up your muscles the way your body is going to use them during your workouts by doing the following series of moves:

- jogging in place (30 seconds)
- walk-outs (30 seconds)
- butt kicks (30 seconds)
- jumping jacks (30 seconds)
- side lunges (30 seconds)
- skipping in place (30 seconds)
- dance! (30 seconds)

You'll do each move in the exact order for thirty seconds each, and that's it! To make things more fun and give your spirit a boost before each workout, here's what I also recommend you try. Pick one killer, four-minute-long song that gets you amped up (I'm talking Taylor Swift or Biggie-caliber music to move your booty to.) That will keep you engaged throughout the entire warmup so you don't slow down at any point and neglect your body in any area.

Finally, why seven moves? Simple! Most trainers would recommend one or two moves to warm up your entire body. But only relying on so few options—such as jogging in place—cheats certain muscles from getting their due. After all, there's not a single exercise that trains your entire body from top to bottom, so why would you rely on *one* exercise to warm up your entire body? That's why my dynamic warmup is a combination of moves that target everything from head to toe.

WHILE YOU LIFT YOURSELF . . .

The way the workout routines are designed, you'll be focusing on either your upper or lower body twice a week. In between you'll specifically target your abs in the middle of the week-long routine.

I can hear you saying, "What? Abs only once?" Don't worry—you'll be working your core muscles every single day, as many of the moves that train your upper and lower body are also core-challenging movements. The reason you'll be doing a core day in the middle is to give your upper and lower body a bit of a break to heal and recover.

The Rules for Each Workout

The basics:

1. Set a timer for twenty-eight minutes, then perform each exercise in the exact order shown in each workout.
2. Once you reach the end of a circuit, rest for sixty seconds. This isn't an active rest, where you're running in between—I want you to take time to recover. So put your hands over your head, take deep breaths, and refocus so you can go hard again immediately afterward.
3. Repeat the circuit once more, and continue to repeat the circuit until your twenty-eight minutes are up.
4. If you reach twenty-eight minutes but haven't performed at least three circuits total, keep moving until you've run through the circuit three times.

Don't sacrifice form for numbers. In my classes I make sure my students go through a complete range of motion and are mindful of how they are performing every exercise rather than having them concentrate on popping out as many repetitions they can as quickly as possible. Doing that only increases your risk of injury and prevents you from getting what you want out of your workout. So with every exercise and stretch, stay focused on how your body needs to move through every repetition and work every muscle through its fullest range of motion.

Tighten your core to LIFT even more. Before each exercise lightly contract your core muscles and try to keep them contracted, no matter which exercise you're doing. Even though many of the moves will engage your core by making your core muscles work behind the scenes to stabilize your body, contracting them at the start helps set the table.

To do it, just pull your navel in toward your spine, then hold it like that. It doesn't have to be extreme. To check yourself, try placing your hand on your stomach and cough. Did you feel what happened to your abs? They should have pulled in to flatten your stomach. That tightness in your midsection should be what you feel before each exercise.

Don't be shocked if you're hungry afterward. When I first started resistance training, I was surprised at how hungry I felt on days when I strength trained. It was this undeniable physiological response that was so different from how my body felt after just going for a run. If that happens to you, just know it's entirely normal.

What you're experiencing is your body breaking down muscle fiber and asking for the proper nutrients to rebuild and come back stronger. In chapter 6 I'll tell you exactly what to eat when that happens, but I just want you to realize and understand why your body's hungry. So if you find yourself hungry after working out, don't be upset. In fact, be thrilled because that's an indicator that you worked your body so sufficiently that it's craving what it needs to repair itself. Good job!

AFTER YOU LIFT YOURSELF . . .
DO THE COOLDOWN

The reason most people dismiss stretching is that they figure it's something only athletes or extremely active people need to do. Not true! Taking a few minutes after your workout to stay limber not only prevents any tightening of certain ligaments and muscles but also helps lower your blood pressure and brings you back to a state of well-being. That's why you'll rely on the following five stretches:

- hamstring stretch
- quad stretch
- the cobra
- chest stretch
- seated glute stretch

You'll do this cooldown at the end of every exercise session, no matter what day it is. Hold each stretch for four or five breaths, then move onto the next stretch—and that's it. There's no need to run through all five a second time, and it should take you no more than two to three minutes. That said, I want you to promise me you won't skip it. Pinky swear to me right now—and remember, *never ever* break a pinky swear promise.

The Routines

Week One

DAY ONE: UPPER BODY

- 10 push-ups
- side plank (right side only) (hold for 30 seconds)
- 10 dips
- mountain climbers (hold for 30 seconds)
- side plank (left side only) (hold for 30 seconds)
- 10 renegade rows (5 each arm)
- high knees (30 seconds)
- 10 up-down planks
- fast feet (30 seconds)
- rest for 60 seconds, then start at the beginning

DAY TWO: LOWER BODY

- 10 glute bridges
- 10 squats
- plank (hold for 30 seconds)
- 20 reverse lunges (10 repetitions each leg)
- wall sits (hold for 30 seconds)
- 10 single-leg Romanian deadlifts (balance on right leg)
- 10 single-leg Romanian deadlifts (balance on left leg)
- 10 burpees
- rest for 60 seconds, then start at the beginning

DAY THREE: ABS

- 10 bird dogs
- plank (hold for 30 seconds)
- high knees (30 seconds)
- Russian twists (30 seconds)
- high knees (30 seconds)
- 10 reach backs (5 each side)
- 4 rock stars (2 each side)
- 10 goddess sit-ups
- fast feet (30 seconds)
- 10 V-ups
- high plank with shoulder taps (30 seconds)
- 10 burpees
- rest for 60 seconds, then start at the beginning

DAY FOUR: CARDIO DAY!

Instead of strength training, you'll be focusing solely on improving your cardiovascular fitness by doing some form of high-intensity interval activity. However, before you start to sweat, you still need to warm up beforehand. Even though whatever cardiovascular exercise you may be doing may not work every muscle in your body from head to toe, it never hurts to have all your muscles warmed up beforehand, so start with the dynamic warm-up. After that you should be good, although it never hurts to do another three to five minutes of whatever activity you're about to do at a low intensity to further warm up your body and make a mind-body connection with what you're about to do.

Once you're set, you have plenty of options to choose from, so pick whichever activity you think you'll put your most heart into:

- Try 30 minutes' worth of sprint intervals: sprint for 30 seconds, then recover for 60 seconds by either walking or putting your hands over your head to refocus so you can go hard again immediately. Repeat 20 times total.
- Take a 30-minute spin class.
- Go for a 30-minute jog: jog for 30 seconds, then walk for 60 seconds. Repeat 20 times total.
- Grab a 30-minute bike ride: either throw it into a high gear or pedal as fast as you can for 30 seconds, then ride at an easy pace for 60 seconds. Repeat 20 times total.
- Do some stairclimbing: run up a flight—or two—of stairs, then walk back down. Repeat 30 minutes total.

If you can't go outside or don't have access to a spin class, stairwell, or stationary equipment, then just sprint in place. That's what we do in my LIFTED classes. In fact, one of the hardest parts of my class is sprinting in place. If you hate to run, you can also use a jump rope or even mimic the movement if you haven't mastered the timing of jumping rope. So long as you're exercising at a high-intensity pace for thirty seconds, then letting yourself recover for one full minute—for thirty straight minutes—then it's all good.

DAY FIVE: UPPER BODY-PLUS

- 10 push-ups
- side plank (right side only) (hold for 30 seconds)
- 10 burpees
- side plank (left side only) (hold for 30 seconds)
- 10 dips
- high planks with shoulder taps (hold for 30 seconds)
- mountain climbers (30 seconds)
- 10 up-down planks
- sumo squat fighters (30 seconds)
- 10 renegade rows (5 each arm)
- speed skaters (30 seconds)
- rest for 60 seconds, then start at the beginning

DAY SIX: LOWER BODY-PLUS

- 10 glute bridges
- 10 single-leg Romanian deadlifts (balance on right leg)
- 10 squats
- 10 single-leg Romanian deadlifts (balance on left leg)
- plank (hold for 30 seconds)
- 10 plyo lunges (right leg only)
- side plank (right side only) (hold for 30 seconds)
- 10 plyo lunges (left leg only)
- side plank (left side only) (hold for 30 seconds)
- 10 drop squats
- fast feet (30 seconds)
- rest for 60 seconds, then start at the beginning

DAY SEVEN: OFF

Week Two

Add either two additional repetitions or five more seconds of time to each exercise. Continue to rest sixty seconds at the end of each circuit.

Week Three

Add another two additional repetitions or five more seconds of time to each exercise. Lower the amount of time you'll rest at the end of each circuit to forty-five seconds instead of sixty.

Week Four

Add another two additional repetitions or five more seconds of time to each exercise. Lower the amount of time you'll rest at the end of each circuit to thirty seconds instead of forty-five.

EXERCISE DESCRIPTIONS

Warm Up

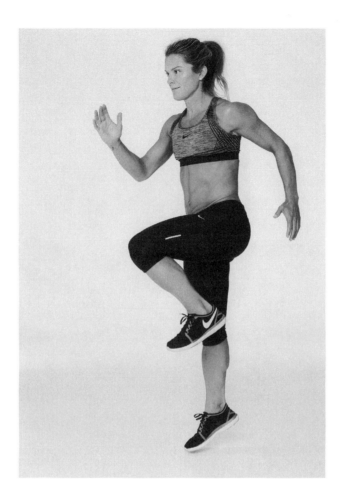

Jogging in Place

GET SET! Stand facing forward with your arms bent at 90-degree angles, forearms parallel to the floor, palms open.

GO! Start jogging in place at a comfortable speed, but pull your knees up high enough so your thighs are almost parallel to the floor. As you jog, pump your arms back and forth and keep your chin up—you should be looking forward the entire time. Continue jogging in place for thirty seconds.

• **Until you're ready to fly!** Try a brisk walk in place instead.

• **Lift yourself higher!** For now don't push this one. This is about getting ready and in the zone. You're stirring up your spirit, so just stay at that pace and be mindful of your movements.

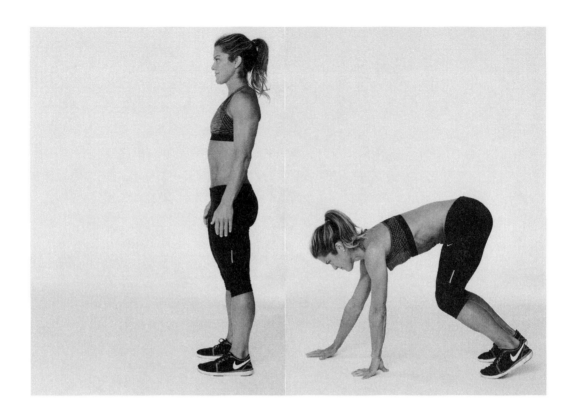

Walk-Outs

GET SET! Stand straight with your feet hip-width apart, with your arms hanging down at your sides.

GO! Bend your knees slightly as you reach down and place your hands shoulder-width apart on the floor. Keeping your feet in place, quickly walk your hands a few inches at a time forward until you're in a push-up position (your body should be one straight line from your head to your heels, with your hands below your shoulders, legs and arms straight, resting on the top of the balls of your feet). Hold this position for one second, then reverse the motion, walking your hands back to return to the GET SET position. Continue doing the move for thirty seconds.

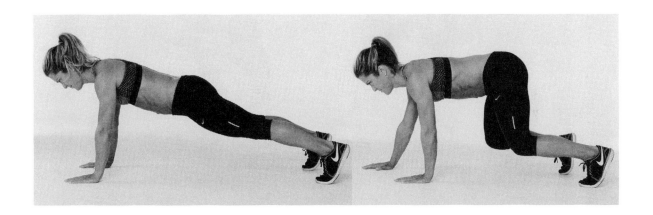

- **Until you're ready to fly!** If you can't get yourself into a push-up position, try going until you're down on all fours. Imagine you're going to look for something on the floor. And don't worry—you'll get there!

- **Lift yourself higher!** For more of a challenge, try to keep your legs straight and bend only at your hips when you begin the exercise. If that's not enough, try walking your hands forward as far as you can instead of stopping when they are directly below your shoulders. This will engage even more of your core.

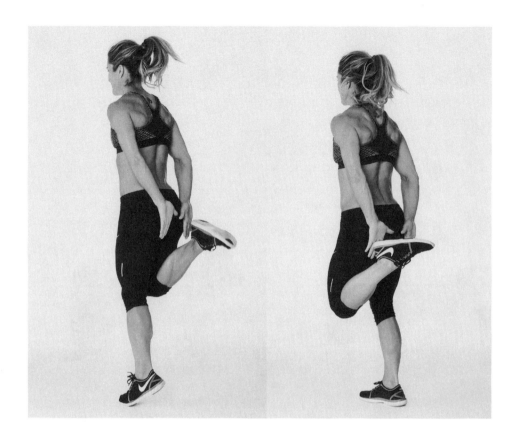

Butt Kicks

GET SET! Stand with your legs together and your arms hanging straight down. Bring your arms back slightly behind you so the backs of your hands are resting on your butt.

GO! Begin by jogging in place. As you go, bring your heel up and back toward your butt so your heels touch the palms of your hands. Continue running in place for thirty seconds.

- **Until you're ready to fly!** If you don't have the flexibility or stamina to get your heel to touch your backside, just try to pull each heel up as high as you can behind you.

- **Lift yourself higher!** Instead of keeping your hands behind you, swing your arms as if you're running to elevate your heart rate even higher.

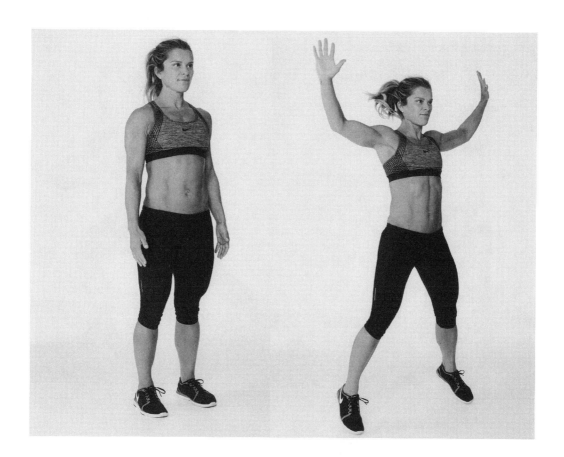

Jumping Jacks

GET SET! Stand facing forward with your arms straight down at your sides.

GO! Bring your arms out from your sides and up as you simultaneously hop high enough to spread your feet wider than shoulder-width apart. Immediately reverse the motion by hopping back into the GET SET position. Repeat the exercise for thirty seconds.

- **Until you're ready to fly!** If thirty seconds is too much, try pausing for one second in between each jumping jack. Or try doing one side at a time, stepping out with your left foot and raising your left arm simultaneously, then doing the same with your right side.

- **Lift yourself higher!** As you do the move, try not to stay in the same position; instead, try turning your body mid-jump and rotate 90 degrees to the left, do a normal jumping jack, then turn your body mid-jump and rotate 90 degrees to the right. Keep alternating back and forth for the duration of the exercise.

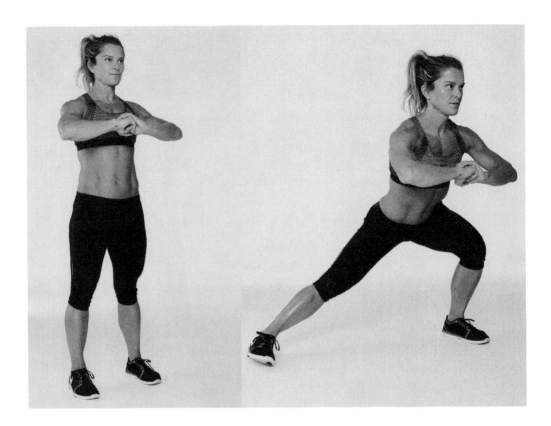

Side Lunge

GET SET! Stand straight with your feet shoulder-width apart. Raise your arms in front of you, make a fist with one hand, and cup your fist with the other. Your forearms should be parallel to the floor, elbows pointing out from your sides.

GO! Keeping your right foot planted, step your left foot out to the left side, push your hips back, and sink into a lunge. Focus on keeping your torso upright and straight as you sit into the lunge, and stop once your left leg is bent at 90 degrees, knee over your toes. Your right leg should end up straight. (Don't worry if your right foot rolls so that you're resting on the inner edge of your right foot. You can't keep it flat on the floor; that's entirely fine.) Reverse the exercise so you're back in the GET SET position, then repeat the move, this time by keeping your left foot planted and stepping your right foot out to your right side. Continue alternating from left to right for thirty seconds.

- **Until you're ready to fly!** If you're having a hard time keeping yourself steady, try extending your arms straight out from your sides for more balance. Or don't come down as far.

- **Lift yourself higher!** At the bottom of the move, try pausing for one second before pushing yourself back up into the GET SET position each time.

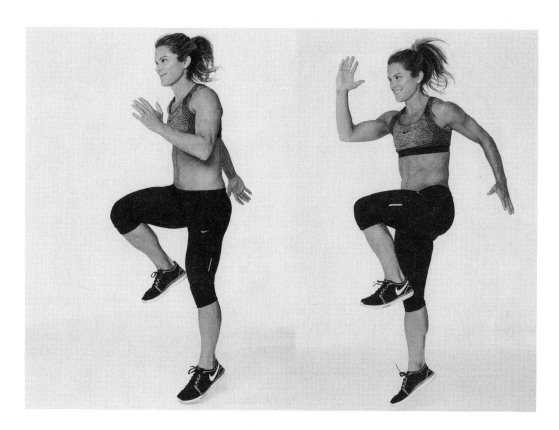

Skipping in Place

GET SET! Stand straight with your arms down by your sides.

GO! Just start skipping at a comfortable pace and try to raise your knees up with each skip as far as you comfortably can. As you go, swing the opposite arm of whichever knee you're raising up in front of you forward.

• **Until you're ready to fly!** If you have a hard time raising your knees as you skip, don't worry about having to lift them up that high as you go.

• **Lift yourself higher!** Because you're still warming, you can try for a little more air time by raising your legs a little bit higher, but don't overdo it.

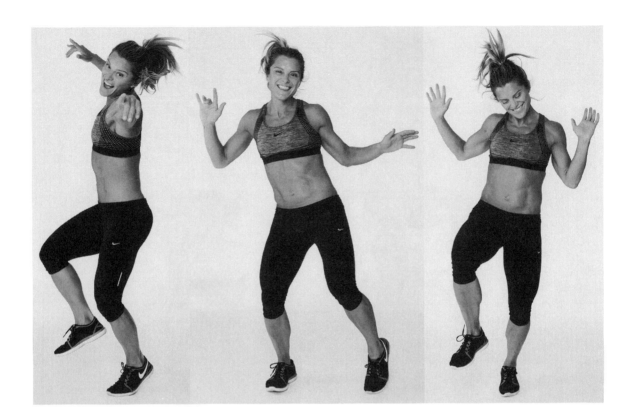

Dancing

GET SET and GO! For this last warmup exercise, just let yourself go and dance any way you like. Pick something playful, and I guarantee that no matter what you choose, you'll target a fair amount of muscles, but more importantly, you'll lift your spirit a little higher and make yourself excited about stepping into your workout. C'mon now! Workouts are supposed to fun, not so serious, so don't look at me like I'm crazy. This is dancing just for yourself, so just let loose a little here, and guess what? You just might surprise yourself!

• **Until you're ready to fly!** If you can't dance, don't worry about it—just move and have fun. Even if you're performing my workout in a gym (or some other place where you may feel too self-conscious to dance), I still encourage you to do it. Why? Because it's a reminder that this is all about you. But if that's simply impossible, I don't want you to interrupt the routine. So if you can't dance, just do the first six warmup exercises for an extra five seconds each when you do them. By doing each move for thirty-five seconds instead of thirty, you'll still wrap up your dynamic warmup in three and a half minutes.

MAIN EXERCISES

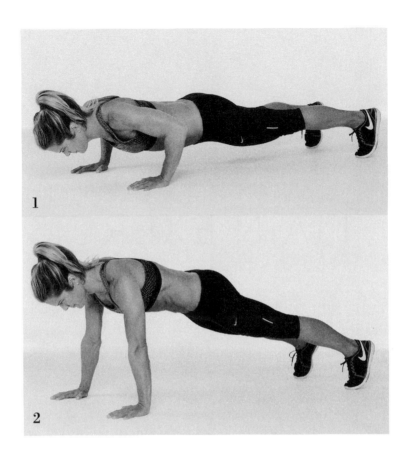

Push-Ups

GET SET! Get into position by placing your hands shoulder-width apart on the floor, then straighten your legs behind you. Straighten your arms to support your weight, with your elbows unlocked. Spread your feet about hip-width apart, and position them so you're resting your weight on your toes and the top of the balls of your feet. Your body should form a straight line from your head to your heels—keep it that way throughout the move.

GO! With your head facing the floor, bend your elbows to lower yourself down toward the floor. You don't have to touch—just stop once your upper arms are parallel to the floor. Immediately press yourself back up by straightening your arms until you're back in the GET SET position.

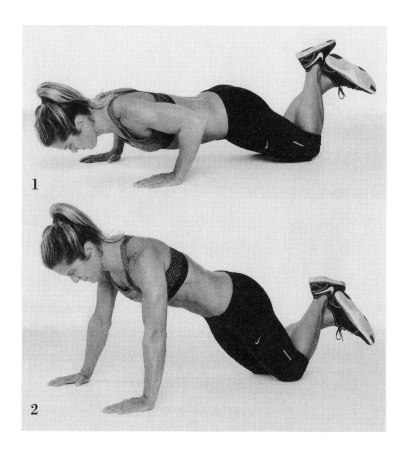

Modified Push-Ups

- **Until you're ready to fly!** If you can't do a push-up yet, try a modified push-up by doing the move with your knees on the ground. Or get into a push-up position and lower yourself down to the ground as slowly as you possibly can. It's okay if you can't push yourself back up; instead, do whatever's necessary to get yourself back into a push-up position. Repeat for the remainder of the exercise.

- **Lift yourself higher!** At the bottom of the exercise, pause for one or two seconds before pressing yourself back up. For an even greater challenge, try taking two to four seconds to lower yourself down, then press yourself back up or try a plyo push-up (press yourself up hard and fast so that your hands leave the floor). As your hands come off, keep your wrists in the same position so you land flat on your palms—not your fingers or knuckles—then immediately sink back down into the next rep.

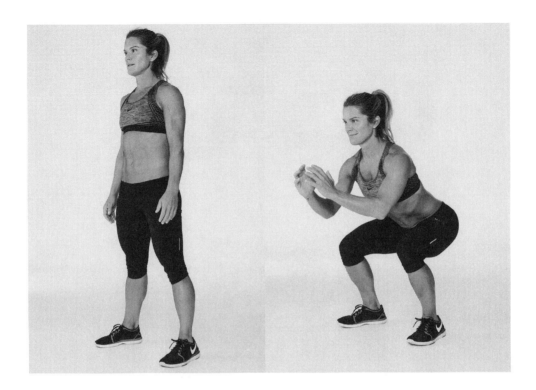

Squats

GET SET! Stand straight with your feet shoulder-width apart, toes pointed slightly outward, and your arms hanging straight down at your sides.

GO! Keeping your head looking forward and your back flat, squat down until your thighs are parallel to the floor, knees in line with your toes (don't let your knees track past your feet). As you drop, bring your arms up in front of you for balance. Pause at the bottom, then press through your heels as you stand back up into the GET SET position. For best results, think about keeping most of your weight on your heels throughout the exercise and pushing through them as you stand back up.

• **Until you're ready to fly!** Instead of squatting down all the way, come down only halfway. Or place a chair behind you so your butt touches down. This will give you a partial rest during each repetition.

• **Lift yourself higher!** There are a lot of different ways to make this move more difficult when you're ready. Try slowing down how quickly you sink into the squat. You can also pause at the bottom of the move for one or two seconds. When even that becomes easy, try holding a pair of dumbbells and keeping your arms either straight down at your sides or, for even more of a challenge, curl the weights up and rest them along the front of your shoulders.

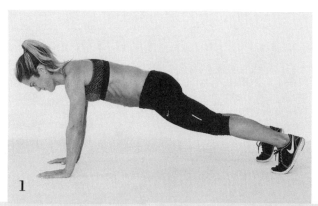

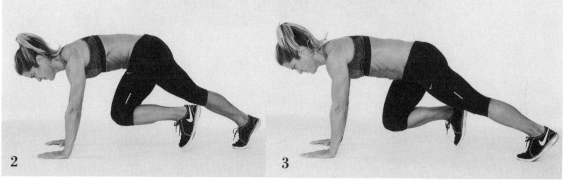

Mountain Climbers

GET SET! Get yourself into the same GET SET position as if you were about to do a push-up. Your hands should be shoulder-width apart and flat on the floor, with your legs extended straight behind you, your weight resting on your toes and the balls of your feet.

GO! Keeping your head facing down to the floor, quickly bring your left knee up toward your chest as far as you comfortably can. Reverse the move to return to the GET SET position, then repeat, this time by quickly bringing your right knee toward your chest. Continue alternating from left to right for the entire exercise. As you go, the exercise should feel as fluid as if you are running.

• **Until you're ready to fly!** If you find it hard to balance or keep the rhythm, just try doing the exercise at a slower pace that's comfortable for you.

• **Lift yourself higher!** Instead of bringing your knee straight up toward your chest underneath you, angle it as you draw it toward your chest so it points to the opposite elbow. For even more of a challenge, try spacing your hands closer together to make it more difficult to balance, or balance yourself on one hand by placing your opposite arm behind your back.

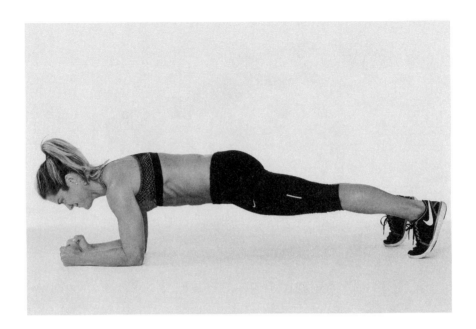

Plank

GET SET! Get yourself into the same GET SET position as if you were about to do a push-up, with your legs extended straight behind you, your weight resting on your toes and the balls of your feet. But instead of placing your hands on the floor, bend your arms and rest on your forearms. Your elbows should be directly below your shoulders, with your head facing down. Finally, pull in your stomach and tighten your core muscles.

GO! Actually, let me rephrase that—STAY! You'll hold this position for the required amount of time. Your body should remain straight. If your hips drop, you'll place too much stress on your lower back. If your butt rises up too far, you'll make the move less effective.

- **Until you're ready to fly!** If you can't hold the position or find yourself breaking form, try a modified plank by starting with your knees on the floor. Or do the move as described for as long as you can, rest for a few seconds, then continue until your time is up.

- **Lift yourself higher!** You can hold the pose for a longer period of time or try raising one foot a few inches off the floor to challenge your stability (just make sure you give equal time to balancing on the opposite leg).

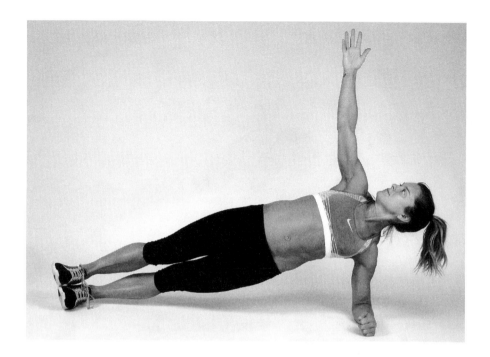

Side Plank

GET SET! Lie down on the floor on your left side with your legs straight and stacked on top of each other. Rest on your left elbow—your left arm should be bent at a 90-degree angle, your elbow below your left shoulder. Extend your right hand up towards the ceiling.

GO! Slowly raise your hips toward the ceiling until your body is perfectly straight from your head down to your feet. Contract your core muscles by bringing your navel in toward your spine. Hold at the top for thirty seconds. Repeat the exercise to work the opposite side of your body.

- **Until you're ready to fly!** Instead of keeping your top hand raised up, try placing it on your hip for balance. If you can't hold yourself up that long, try a modified version of the side plank. To do it, stay in the same position, only bend your legs so your feet are behind you. Your legs should be bent at a 90-degree angle.

- **Lift yourself higher!** If that's still too easy, keep your nonworking arm raised, but try holding a light dumbbell when you do it. Or try raising whichever leg is on top up toward the ceiling and hold it in that position as you perform the move.

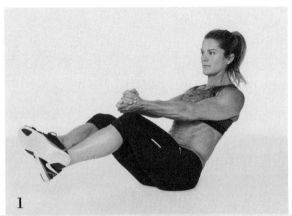

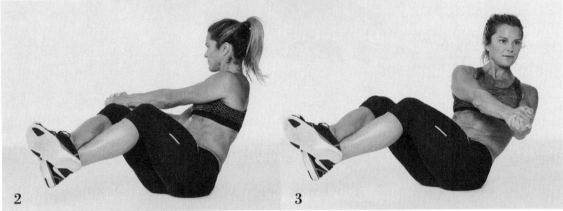

Russian Twists

GET SET! Sit on the floor with your knees bent, feet crossed, and your heels raised off the floor. Straighten your arms out in front of you, and clasp your hands, then slowly lean back until your torso is at a 45-degree angle. You should be balancing on just your butt.

GO! Keeping your arms straight and feet raised on the floor, slowly rotate to the right as far as you can without losing your balance. Return to the GET SET position, then repeat the move by slowly rotating to the left. Keep alternating back and forth throughout the exercise for the required amount of time.

- **Until you're ready to fly!** If you can't keep your balance, place your feet flat on the floor about shoulder width apart.

- **Lift yourself higher!** Hold a light dumbbell or a medicine ball with both hands to add more weight to the move.

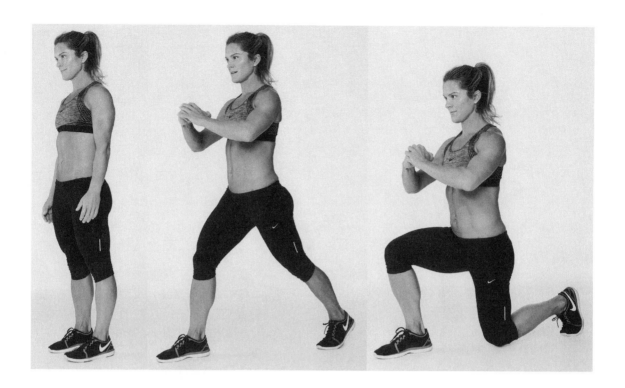

Reverse Lunges

GET SET! Stand straight with your feet hip-width apart. Raise your arms in front of you, make a fist with one hand, and cup your fist with the other, with elbows pointing out from your sides.

GO! Take a big step backward with your left foot, and lower yourself down by bending your right knee until your right thigh is parallel to the floor. Your left knee should almost graze the floor—but don't let it touch. Your goal should be to have both legs bent at 90-degree angles. Push yourself back up into the GET SET position, then repeat, this time stepping back with your right leg. Continue to alternate from left to right for the duration of the exercise.

- **Until you're ready to fly!** If you can't lunge all the way down, place a chair alongside yourself and grab it for balance as you perform the exercise.

- **Lift yourself higher!** Try adding a little weight to the move by holding a pair of dumbbells. You can either hold them with your arms down by your sides, curl them up so they are positioned in front of your shoulders, or if you're ready for a real challenge, try keeping them pressed above your head as you go.

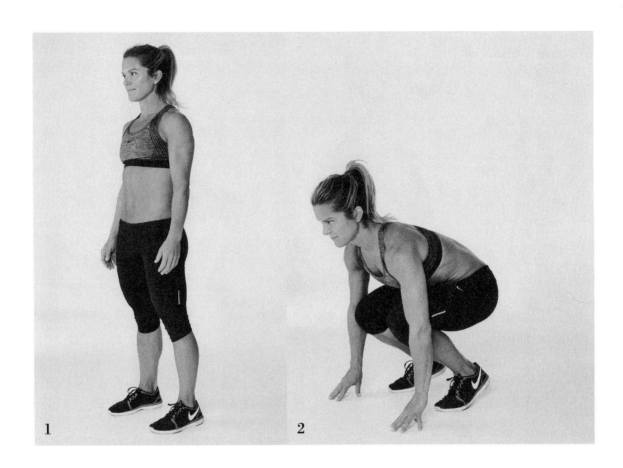

Burpees

GET SET! Stand straight with your feet hip-width apart and your arms hanging straight down from your sides.

GO! Quickly bend down and place your hands flat on the floor, then immediately shoot your legs straight behind you so you end up in the top portion of a push-up. Bend your elbows, and drop your body to the floor. Then, without pausing, push yourself up, and immediately jump your feet forward so they land between your hands. Finally, quickly jump up as high as you can with your arms extended above your head. As you land, immediately repeat the exercise by bending down and putting your hands flat on the floor. The move should be continuous—think: squat, push-up and jump—so don't stop.

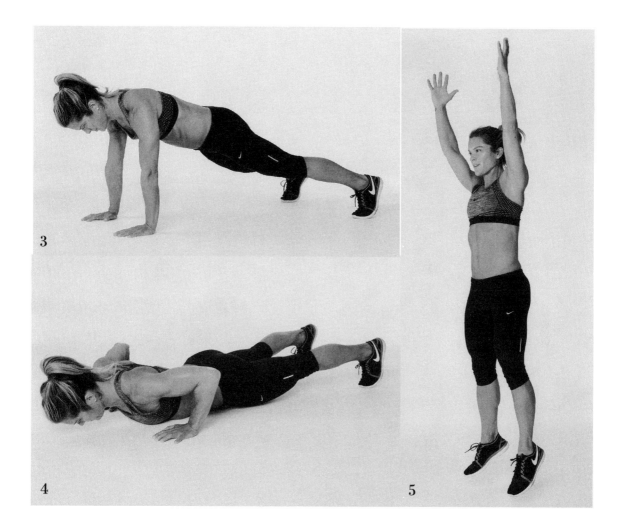

- **Until you're ready to fly!** You can make this easier several ways. After you land, pause for a moment each time before continuing the exercise. Or skip the jumping part entirely and simply stand up for each repetition. Finally, instead of thrusting your legs back and/or jumping them forward, try stepping them forward or backward instead.

- **Lift yourself higher!** There are several ways to add more intensity to this already intense exercise. As you jump up, try turning in midair 180 degrees so you land in the opposite direction, or try tucking your knees up toward your chest.

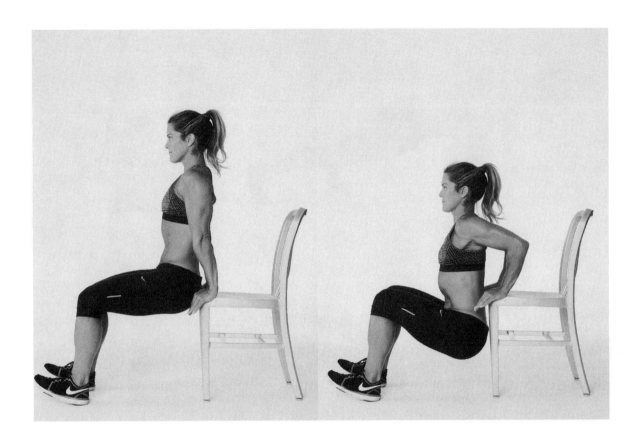

Dips

GET SET! Sit on the edge of a sturdy chair with your hands on the chair, palms down alongside your hips, knuckles facing forward. Shimmy your butt forward and off the seat until you're supporting your body weight with your arms. Your knees should be bent with your feet on the floor, heels down and toes up.

GO! Without moving your feet, slowly bend your elbows and lower your butt down toward the floor until your arms are bent at a 90-degree angle. Your body should stay as close to the chair as possible as you go. Slowly press yourself back up into the GET SET position until your arms are straight, elbows unlocked.

· **Until you're ready to fly!** If you can't drop all the way down, just lower yourself about halfway.

· **Lift yourself higher!** Position another chair across from you and place your feet on top of that instead. Or get a friend to place a light medicine ball or dumbbell on top of your thighs.

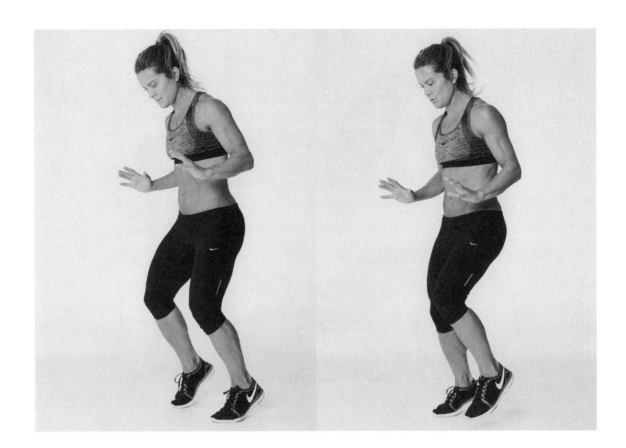

Fast Feet

GET SET! Stand with your feet a few inches apart and up on the balls of your feet, heels raised. Your arms should be bent at 90 degrees, elbows tucked into your sides, with your palms facing down.

GO! Keeping your heels raised and arms up, step your feet up and down as quickly as you can—left foot, right foot. Don't raise your feet any higher than an inch from the floor—this move is about moving as quickly as possible, not lifting yourself any higher than you need to.

- **Until you're ready to fly!** Try the exercise at a slower pace.

- **Lift yourself higher!** Perform the exercise at full intensity, but extend your arms out to the sides with one arm up and one arm down. As you move your feet, quickly move your arms at the same time so that one is always down and the other is always up. Imagine someone is trying to get a ball past you, and you want to block the shot. Or if you have the space, try moving yourself both forward and backward as you go.

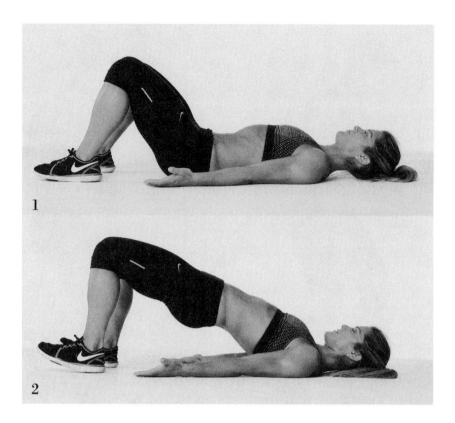

Glute Bridges

GET SET! Lie flat on your back with your knees bent and your feet flat on the floor spaced hip-width apart. Position your arms down by your sides with your palms facing up.

GO! Without moving your arms, press down through your heels and contract your glutes (your butt muscles) as you raise your hips up. Stop once your body forms a straight line from your knees to your neck. Squeeze your glutes for a second, then lower your butt back down to the floor.

- **Until you're ready to fly!** If you need more stability, try extending your arms out to your sides with your palms facing down. If you have a difficult time raising your hips as high, just raise them as far as you comfortably can.

- **Lift yourself higher!** Instead of having your butt touch down after every repetition, let it hover about an inch off the ground each time to keep constant tension on your muscles. Or you can place your heels on a sturdy box or object that's between eighteen to twenty-four inches high, which will change the angle of the exercise. Finally, instead of keeping both feet on the floor, extend one leg straight out at a 45-degree angle, then keep it in that position as you go up and down (just make sure you give the opposite leg equal attention so your muscles stay balanced).

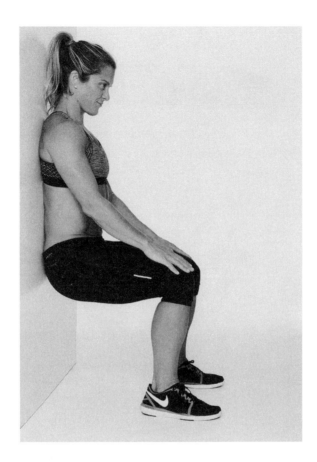

Wall Sits

GET SET! Find a sturdy wall, and stand with your back facing it, about two feet away from it. Space your feet shoulder-width apart, with your toes slightly pointing outward. Rest yourself on the wall so your head and back are flat against it, then lower yourself until your thighs are parallel to the floor. Finally, place your arms out in front of you, palms on your legs.

GO! Actually, I want you to stay. Hold this position without moving for the required period of time.

• **Until you're ready to fly!** Try going down halfway, or do the exercise as described for as long as you can, stand back up to take a few seconds breather, then sink back down into position until your time is up.

• **Lift yourself higher!** Once you're in the GET SET position, try raising one foot an inch off the floor and hold it there for half the time (make sure to do it with the opposite foot for the back half of the exercise so your muscles are worked evenly).

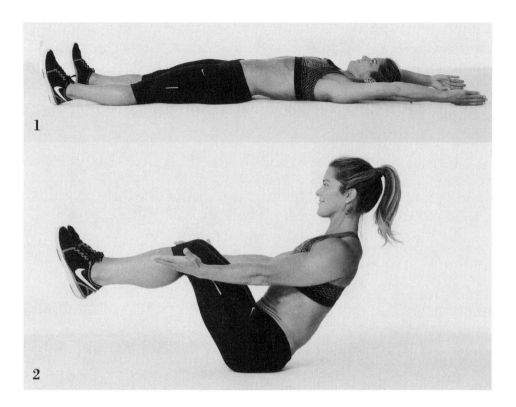

V-Ups

GET SET! Lie flat on your back with your legs straight and your arms down by your sides.

GO! Keeping your back flat, simultaneously raise your knees and torso up so they are both at a 45-degree angle (your thighs and torso from the side should look like the letter V). As you rise, extend your arms forward, pointing your hands toward your feet. Reverse the motion by lowering yourself back down to the floor to return to the GET SET position.

• **Until you're ready to fly!** If you find it hard to balance or lack the core strength to come all the way up, just raise your legs and torso as high as you comfortably can.

• **Lift yourself higher!** There are many options you can try: in the up position, pause, then rotate from your waist to the left, then to the right, before lowering yourself back down each time. For more of a challenge, start the move with your arms extended alongside your head, then sweep them forward as you do the move. You can even add resistance by holding a light medicine ball or dumbbell.

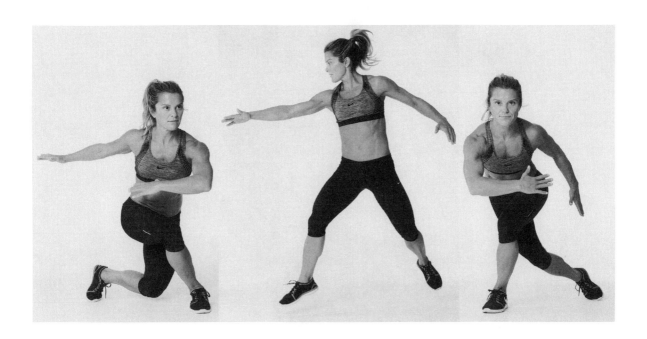

Speed Skaters

GET SET! Stand straight, with your feet hip-width apart and your arms down by your sides.

GO! Keeping your body facing forward, quickly leap to your right side by pushing off with your left foot. Land on your right foot, and let your left leg sweep behind you as if you were skating. Quickly jump to the left by pushing off your right foot. Land on your left foot, and let your right leg sweep back behind you. Keep jumping back and forth for the required number of repetitions.

I love this move! Talk about getting LIFTED! I feel like I can fly with this move, and it always shakes up my spirit. So throw that arm out to the side and SOAR!

- **Until you're ready to fly!** Each time you land, let the foot of your back leg touch the floor for a second or two to give you a breather.

- **Lift yourself higher!** Each time you land, bend down and touch the floor with the hand opposite of the leg you're balancing on—for example, if you're balancing on your left leg, touch the floor with the right hand, and vice versa.

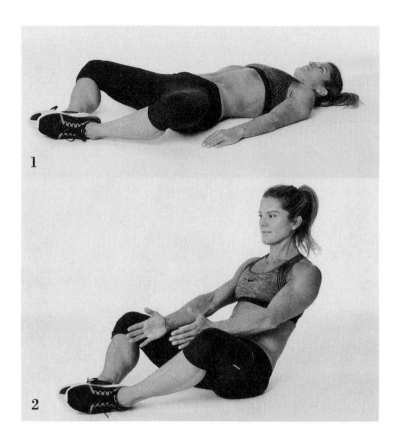

Goddess Sit-Ups

GET SET! Lie flat on your back with your arms straight down at your sides, palms down. Place the soles of your feet together so your knees point out to the sides—this helps release your psoas, the deep muscle that connects your spine to your legs.

GO! Keeping the soles of your feet together, contract your core muscles, then slowly curl your head, shoulders, and back off the floor as you extend your arms forward toward your feet. Stop when your back is about a 45-degree angle from the floor, then lower yourself back down into the GET SET position.

• **Until you're ready to fly!** Instead of placing the soles of your feet together, just perform a normal crunch. Start with your knees bent, feet flat on the floor, and your hands lightly touching behind your ears. Crunch up by raising your head and shoulders off the floor, then lower yourself back down.

• **Lift yourself higher!** Start with your arms extended behind you, then sweep them up and forward as you perform the move. For even more of a challenge, hold a light medicine ball or dumbbell with both hands.

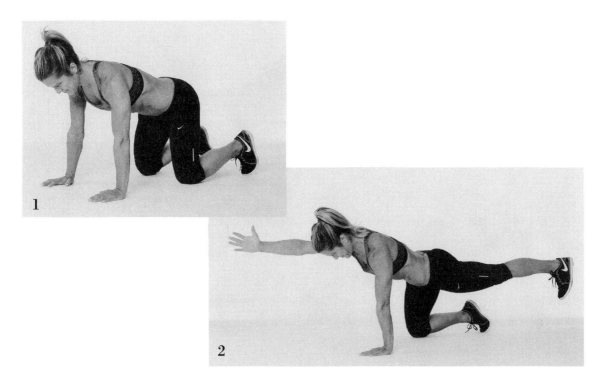

Bird Dogs

GET SET! Get on the floor on your hands and knees, with your hands positioned directly below your shoulders and your knees directly below your hips. Keep your neck straight, your head in line with your spine, facing down toward the floor, and your core muscles tight.

GO! Maintaining your balance, extend your right arm straight out in front of you as you simultaneously extend your left leg straight back. Resist the urge to look upward—your head should stay in line with your spine. Pause for one second at the top, return to the GET SET position, and repeat the exercise, this time by extending your left arm straight out in front and extend your right leg straight back. Continue to alternate for the duration of the exercise.

- **Until you're ready to fly!** Instead of extending one arm and one leg simultaneously, try doing one at a time.

- **Lift yourself higher!** Once you're in the extended position—one arm and one leg straightened out—instead of just placing them back on the floor, try drawing your elbow and knee toward each other under your body until they touch. Then extend your arm and leg out once more, then put them on the floor. Or instead of starting the exercise on your knees, get into a push-up position and perform the move—you'll find this challenges your balance even more.

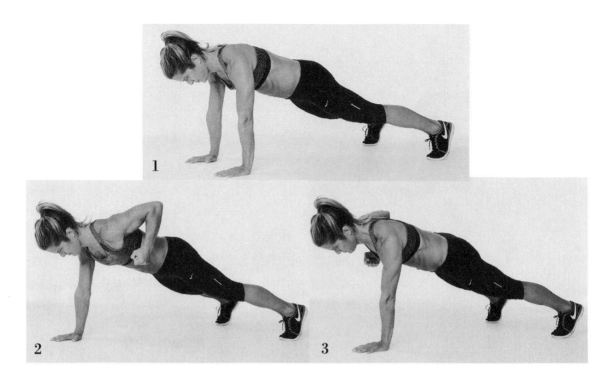

Renegade Row

GET SET! Get yourself into the same GET SET position as if you were about to do a push-up. Your hands should be shoulder-width apart and flat on the floor, with your legs extended straight behind you, your weight resting on your toes and the balls of your feet. Finally, space your feet out slightly wider than shoulder-width apart for stability.

GO! Maintaining your balance, shift your weight onto your right hand as you bend your left arm, and row your left fist up as high as you comfortably can. Lower your left arm back into the GET SET position, then repeat the exercise, this time shifting your weight onto your right hand and raising your right fist up as high as you can. Continue alternating from left to right for the entire exercise.

- **Until you're ready to fly!** The farther your feet are apart, the more of a base you'll have to maintain your balance, so try widening your stance. If the move is still too difficult, pull your arm up only about half the distance.

- **Lift yourself higher!** Try spacing your feet closer together or right next to each other. If that's still too easy, try pausing at the top of the move for at least two seconds, or add some weight by using a pair of dumbbells.

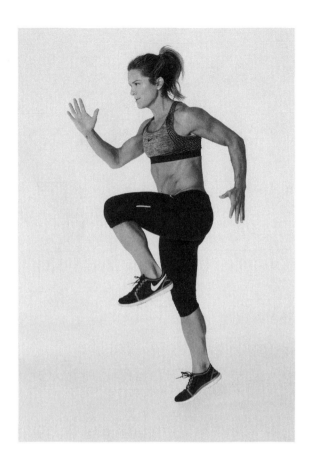

High Knee Sprints

GET SET! Stand straight, with your arms hanging down from your sides.

GO! Begin sprinting at a fast pace. As you go, try to bring each knee up as high as possible toward your chest. Swing whichever arm is opposite the knee you're raising forward to help you build momentum.

Something about this move makes me feel like I'm chasing down my dreams. I tell my students that you're either running away from something—or toward something. It's always sweeter to run toward something, so envision something you want to chase down with this move.

- **Until you're ready to fly!** Either lower the speed or just raise your knees as far as you comfortably can.

- **Lift yourself higher!** Try to up the intensity by moving as fast as you can, as if you were seconds from crossing a finish line.

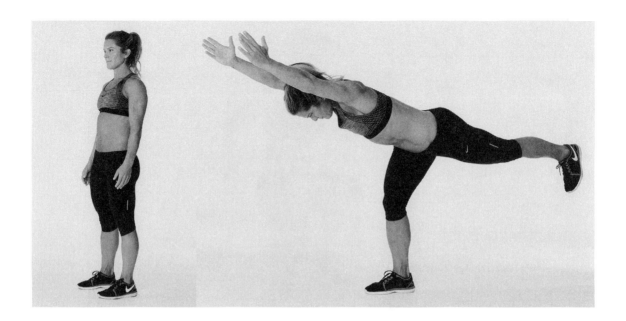

Single-Leg Romanian Deadlifts

GET SET! Stand straight, with your arms down by your sides.

GO! Shift your weight onto your right leg, and lift your left foot slightly off the ground behind you. Maintaining your balance, push your hips back as far as you can to lower your torso toward the floor, keeping your back flat, while reaching forward with both hands. Your left leg should naturally swing straight back behind you. Squeeze your glutes to raise yourself back in the GET SET position. Repeat the exercise on your right leg for the required number of repetitions. Change positions to work your left leg.

When we do this move in my classes, I watch people lose their balance for the first few repetitions all the time. That's why I tell them to move with *grace!* Even if you don't think you *have* grace, pretend like you do. Reach your hands forward with elegance and grace, and see how much better you do!

- **Until you're ready to fly!** Instead of completely raising your back leg as high as possible behind you, go only as far as you can, and touch your back foot to the floor behind you to regain stability. Another tip to try: focus on a spot in front of you or on the floor that can help steady you. If it's still a challenge, just do your best and know this: you're going to get better, so don't beat yourself up for being a little wobbly for now.

- **Lift yourself higher!** To add more to the exercise, try holding a pair of dumbbells, but don't extend your arms when you do the exercise—just let them hang straight down throughout the entire move so you don't strain your back.

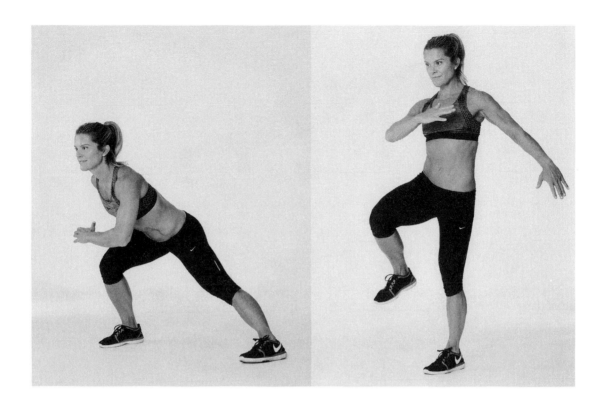

Plyo Side Lunge

(Just so you know, this exercise is a modified version of the side lunge on page 66, only you'll be explosively pushing yourself up instead of gently returning to the GET SET position.)

GET SET! Stand straight, with your feet hip-width apart and your arms down by your sides. (By the way, don't worry about your arms throughout the exercise; just let them swing naturally as you go.)

GO! Keeping your left leg planted, step your right foot out to the right side, and shift your weight onto your right foot. Your left leg should end up straight (don't worry if your left foot rolls so that you're resting on the inner edge of your left foot). Quickly and powerfully push yourself back up toward center, and balance only on your left foot, then immediately step to the side again with your right leg. Continue lunging with your right leg for the required number of repetitions. (To do your left leg, just reverse direction.)

- **Until you're ready to fly!** If you can't put much force into the move, just do a normal side lunge (see description on page 66). Or each time you land, instead of balancing on one foot, allow your other foot to touch down to temporarily give your muscles a break.

- **Lift yourself higher!** Try holding a medicine ball with both hands in front of your chest.

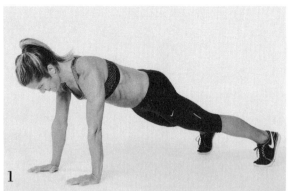

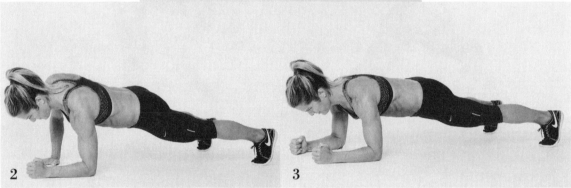

Up-Down Plank

GET SET! Get down on the floor in a push-up position, with your hands shoulder-width apart and your legs extended behind you, feet also shoulder-width apart.

GO! While maintaining your balance, bend your left arm, and place your left forearm on the floor, then do the same with your right arm—you should be resting on both forearms with your elbows directly below your shoulders. Immediately reverse the exercise—left arm first, then your right—until you're back in the GET SET position. That's one repetition. Repeat the exercise, but this time let your right arm bend first, then your left. Keep switching from left to right for the entire exercise.

- **Until you're ready to fly!** Instead of doing the exercise with your legs straight, keep your knees on the floor.

- **Lift yourself higher!** Try raising one foot off the floor behind you and keeping it there for half of the repetitions. Then raise the opposite foot off the floor for the remainder of the exercise.

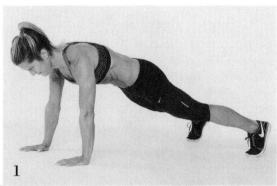

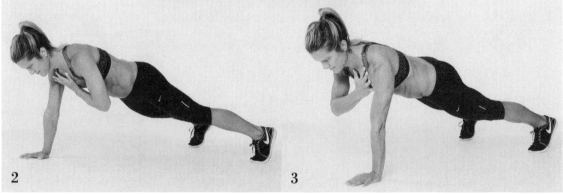

High Plank with Shoulder Tap

GET SET! Get down on the floor in a push-up position, with your hands shoulder-width apart and your legs extended behind you, feet also shoulder-width apart.

GO! Maintaining your balance, shift your weight onto your right arm, then reach up with your left hand and touch your right shoulder. Place your hand back on the floor and repeat, this time shifting your weight onto your left arm and reaching up with your right hand to touch your

left shoulder. Continue alternating back and forth for the duration of the exercise. As you go, don't allow your body to twist—your hips should remain square to the floor at all times.

• **Until you're ready to fly!** If you find it hard to maintain your balance, try the exercise with your knees on the ground.

• **Lift yourself higher!** To make the move more difficult, try doing it as slowly as possible.

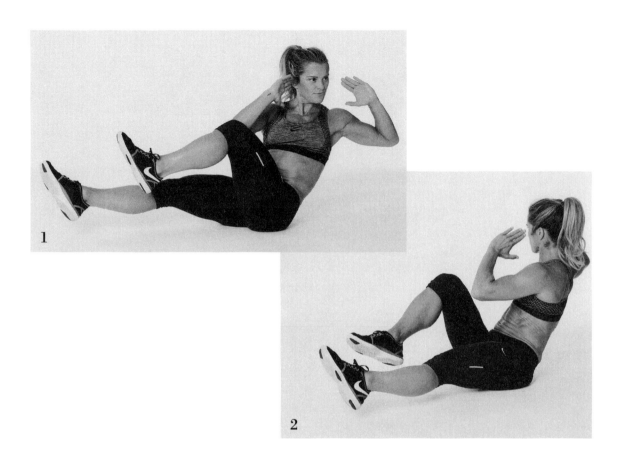

Slow Bicycles

GET SET! Lie on the floor with your legs bent, arms bent behind your head, and your hands framing your face. Your elbows should be pointing out from your sides. Raise your head and shoulders just off the floor.

GO! Begin cycling by slowly pulling your left knee in toward your chest as you extend your right leg forward, keeping it suspended just off the floor. Simultaneously curl your torso up, and twist to your left and touch your right elbow to your left knee (or at least get them close to each other). Slowly reverse the motion, this time drawing your right knee in to meet your left elbow as you twist to the right. Continue to alternate from left to right, keeping your feet off the floor the entire time. Don't rush the move: each leg should take you a count of two seconds.

- **Until you're ready to fly!** Try doing the move at a faster pace, or let your feet touch the floor each time you extend your leg to give your core muscles a breather.

- **Lift yourself higher!** Instead of taking two seconds per leg, try to slow the move down even further and make it three to four seconds.

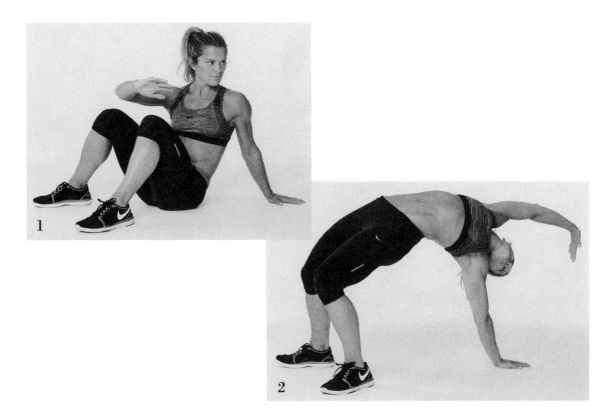

Rock Stars

GET SET! Sit on the floor with your legs bent, feet flat, shoulder-width apart. Reach your left arm back behind you, shift your weight to your left hip, and place your left hand flat on the floor. Bend your right arm, and position it in front of you.

GO! Keeping your left hand on the floor, gently push your hips up toward the ceiling as you extend your right arm straight up. Continue arching your back as you drop your head and right arm behind you as far as you comfortably can. Pause for a second, and squeeze your glutes, then return to the GET SET position, and change positions to work the other side of your body—this time by placing your right arm behind you as you reach up and back with your left arm.

When I do this move in my classes, everybody loves it because it makes you feel so elegant and powerful. So expect to feel like a rock star. And when you do it, I want you to really own it!

- **Until you're ready to fly!** If you don't have the flexibility to fully arch your back, just raise your hips up as high as you can.

- **Lift yourself higher!** To enhance this pose, try holding the top position for three to four seconds.

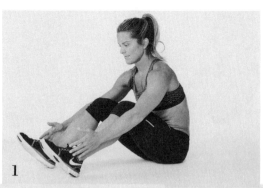

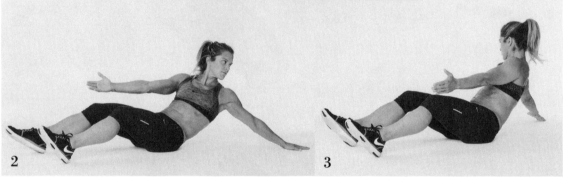

Reach Backs

GET SET! Begin by sitting on the floor with your legs bent in front of you, toes raised and heels on the floor. Straighten your arms in front of you, aiming your fingers toward your feet.

GO! With your core muscles braced for stability, keep your right arm pointing forward as you lean back and reach behind yourself as far as possible with your left hand. Try to stay focused on staying balanced on your butt as you go. Touch the floor with your left hand, then bring yourself back to the GET SET position. Repeat the exercise again, only this time keep your left arm pointed forward as you reach back with your right hand.

• **Until you're ready to fly!** If you're having a hard time balancing, try bending your legs more so your feet remain flat on the floor. If that's still difficult, try placing the hand of whichever arm is pointing forward as you lean back on your leg.

• **Lift yourself higher!** To really challenge your core muscles, try keeping your heels elevated above the floor no more than an inch throughout the entire exercise.

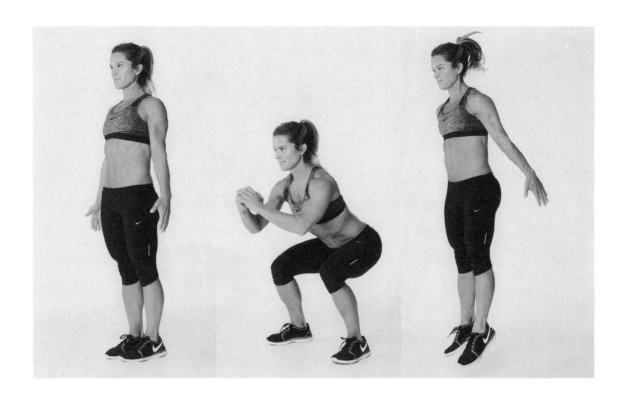

Drop Squats

GET SET! Stand straight, with your feet together and your arms down by your sides.

GO! Quickly hop your feet out about shoulder-width apart as you simultaneously sink into a squat, swinging your arms forward as you go so your hands end up in front of you, elbows bent. Immediately jump straight up as you swing your arms back behind you and bring your feet together. Land in the GET SET position, and repeat for the required number of repetitions.

I feel like I'm dancing with this move. I touch my hand to the ground, and then elevate! This is a great move to match the rhythm of the music, so even though I've never been a dancer, I act like and *believe* I am one when I do this exercise! **So really let yourself GO!**

- **Until you're ready to fly!** Instead of quickly hopping your feet out each time you squat, just step your feet out so they're shoulder-width apart. To give yourself a breather, you can always pause for one second in the GET SET position before continuing the exercise.

- **Lift yourself higher!** Instead of landing with your legs together, quickly click your heels together, then space your feet shoulder-width apart before you land. Once you do, immediately sink right back into the squat position.

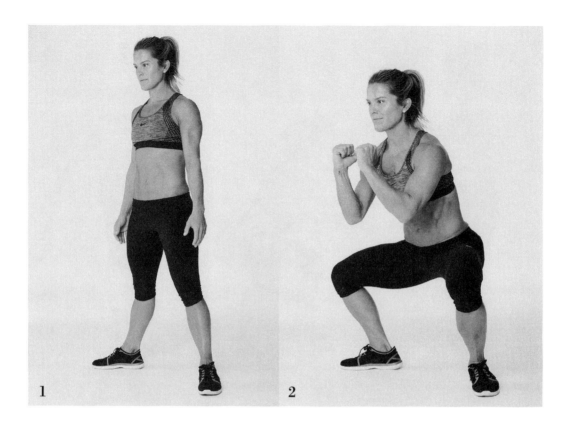

1

2

Sumo Squat Fighter

GET SET! Stand with your arms down to your sides and your feet spaced wider than shoulder-width apart, toes angled out.

Before you try it, remember this: it's time to wake up the fight in you! This a great opportunity to let go of any tension and punch away anything that's just not worthy of your day!

GO! Lower yourself into a squat position until your thighs are parallel to the floor. As you drop, bend your arms, and bring your fists just below your chin, elbows bent and pointed toward the floor. Quickly punch your left fist across your body to your right side, then bring your left fist back into position as you quickly punch your right fist across your body to your left side. Bring your fists just below your chin once again, then stand up. That's one repetition.

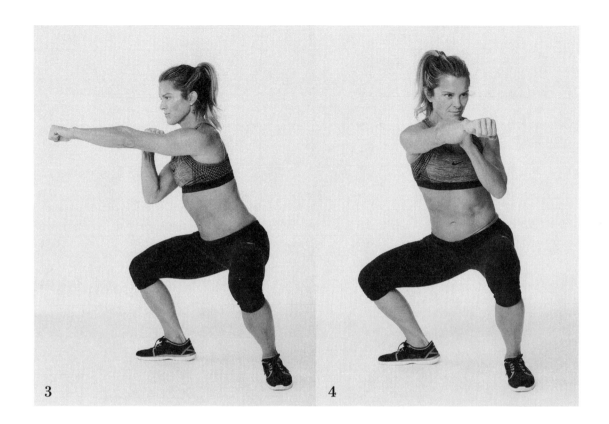

Tip: Don't twist at the waist. Even though your torso will rotate slightly as you do the move, this move is an antirotational exercise. The object is to keep your body from rotating, which will challenge your core muscles naturally as you punch.

- **Until you're ready to fly!** Instead of doing four repetitions, try doing two to three.

- **Lift yourself higher!** Instead of doing four repetitions, try doing six to eight.

COOL-DOWN MOVES

Stretch

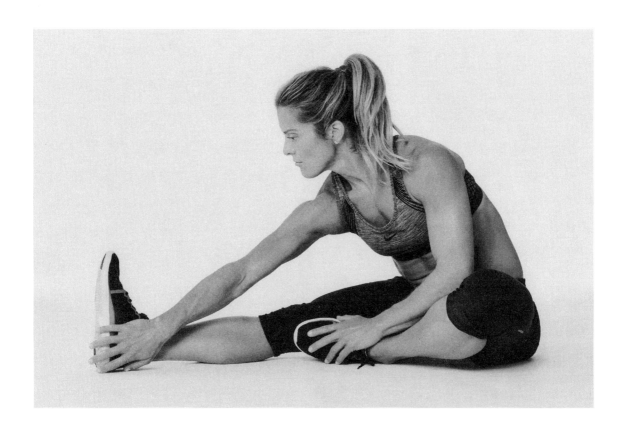

Hurdler Stretch

Stretches: the hamstrings (the muscles along the back of your thighs), low back, and calves.

GET SET! Sit down on the floor and straighten your right leg out in front of you. Bend your left knee, and place the sole of your left foot along the inside of your right leg.

GO! Slowly bend at the waist, and grab your right foot with your right hand—if you're not that flexible, just try to grab as far down your leg as you can. You can rest your left hand wherever is comfortable. Hold for about four to five deep breaths, then switch legs.

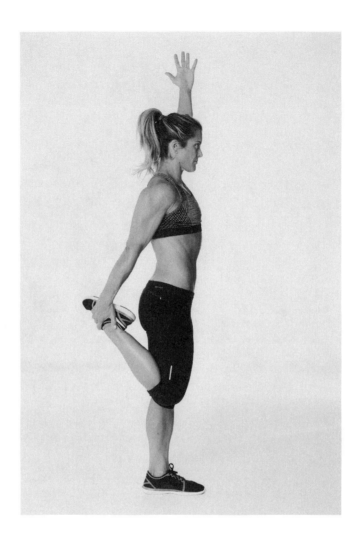

Quadriceps Stretch

Stretches: the quadriceps (the muscles along the front of your thighs).

GET SET! Bend your right knee, and raise your right foot up behind you toward your butt, then reach back and grab it with your right hand. Extend your left arm up toward the ceiling.

GO! Gently use your right hand to pull your right heel in toward your butt as far as you comfortably can. Hold for about four to five deep breaths, then gently place your foot back down to the floor. Switch positions to stretch your left leg, this time grabbing your left foot with your left hand and extending your right arm up toward the ceiling.

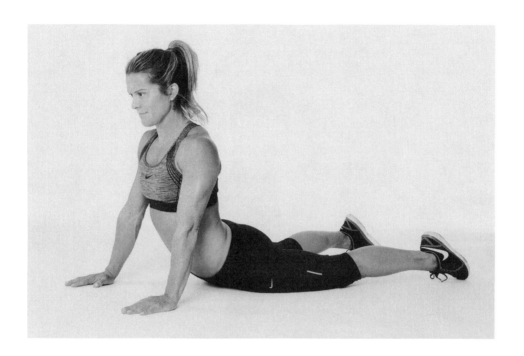

The Cobra

Stretches: the abdominals and spine.

GET SET! Lie flat on your stomach, with your hands flat on the ground, palms directly beneath your shoulders. Your legs should be straight, with the tops of your feet flat on the floor.

GO! Slowly lift your chest up off the ground by straightening your arms, keeping your legs and hips flat on the floor. Hold for about four to five deep breaths, then lower yourself back down to the floor.

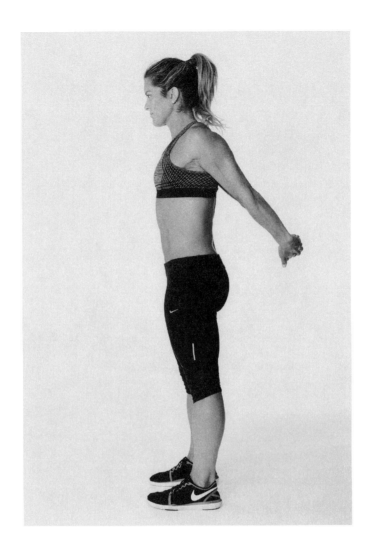

Chest Stretch

Stretches: the chest and shoulders.

GET SET! Stand with your feet shoulder-width apart and your arms down by your sides. Reach your arms back behind you, and interlace your hands together, palms facing toward you.

GO! Keeping your arms straight and fingers interlaced, gently raise your arms upward as far as you comfortably can, and hold for about four to five deep breaths.

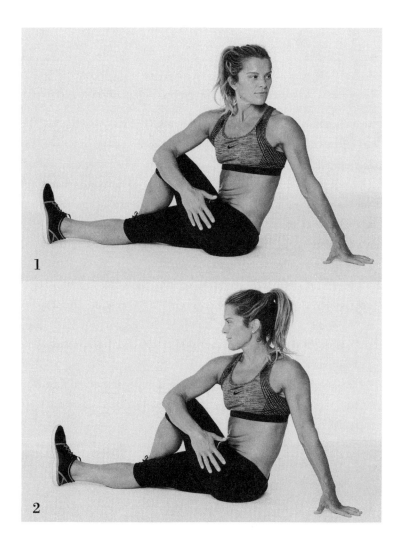

Seated Glute Stretch

Stretches: the glutes and hips.

GET SET! Sit down on the floor and straighten your legs out in front of you. Bend your left leg, and drop your left foot down on the floor on the opposite side of your right leg.

GO! Wrap your right arm around the outside of your left knee, clasp your hands, and gently pull your left knee in toward your body until you feel a comfortable stretch in your hips and glutes. Hold for about four to five deep breaths, then switch positions to stretch the right side of your body.

Weave Music into Your Workout

Music is a huge part of how I teach, and I'm very particular about which songs I select—as well as their arrangement—because I need to LIFT fifty people up at one time. In my classes we actually move to the rhythm of the music not just because it lifts their spirits and motivates them but because it forces them to work through a greater range of motion. That's why—if you're looking to up your game—I encourage you to consider thinking ahead of time about creating a hit list of songs that could lift you up even higher when you're working out.

There's no *right* way to do it, so long as what you pull together is at least twenty-eight minutes long and has a motivating effect on your spirit.

- You might do it in a way that builds you up, then brings you down in a positive way.
- You might choose songs by how many beats per minute (for strength training, any songs between 130 and 140 beats per minute is usually best).
- You might even do it chronologically so that the music takes you on a journey throughout your life or stops at a specific time in your life when you found the greatest inspiration.

But if you have no idea where to start, that's fine too. Allow *me* to LIFT you! You'll find a few of my favorite playlists that work perfectly with each workout at Spotify—just link to my account (Holly Rilinger).

Even I Was LIFTED Later in Life . . .

It may surprise you, but it took me many years to recognize that strength training changes your body in a different way than cardio does. I used to be a cardio junkie, and when I was training specifically for basketball, I ran through a lot of court-specific drills that were all about performance. None of those drills were ever about body image.

Then when I stopped playing basketball, I started training myself—and I exercised much like most women do. I would go out and run for an hour because exercise was all about how many calories I could burn. I didn't understand the science of strength training and how it was critical to keeping me fitter and leaner. It was a screwed-up way to think, and I don't know how so many of us got into this mess of doing too much cardio and thinking we need to starve ourselves to lose body fat—but somehow we did.

It wasn't until I became a trainer that I started to educate myself and study anatomy and physiology within the gym model. That's when I began to understand how having less muscle causes your metabolism to slow down, burn fewer calories, and store remaining calories as unwanted fat. That's when I learned that adding some form of regular resistance training could raise your metabolism by as much as 15 percent.[1]

But that's also when I connected with how regular resistance training also makes you less likely to have metabolic syndrome, a group of five risk factors—from having a large waist to high blood pressure—that have been proven to increase your risk of developing diabetes and heart disease. Again, you might have chosen LIFTED to change your body—and it will—but know that you'll be changing it in ways that go much farther than just how it looks. Believe me and trust the process—it won't let you fall.

4

Spirit (AKA Smile!)

It's not until you come to a place of gratitude that you can ever truly change a thing about yourself. And it's not until you recognize that lifting your spirit is equally as important as lifting your mind and body that you'll ever be able to spread your wings and SOAR.

It's what I believe in, how I live my life, and the lasting imprint I want to leave on every person who walks into my life—whether it's the students in my classes or someone I meet while grabbing coffee. And that includes *you*!

That's why at the end of each LIFTED class I ask everyone to lie back and have a moment of surrender, with their arms falling at their sides as they let it all go. For me song selection is *everything* in this moment, and I always choose something that speaks to my *soul*!

Even though this moment is mostly about letting the last hour of exercise sink in along with letting go of anything that's not coming with them, it's also when I touch upon some very simple things, things I believe are tools and sound bites they can take with them to help them appreciate what they've accomplished.

I may talk about how our day felt so far away from us over the last forty-five minutes, where we let go of the things that weren't worthy of our day. I may remind them that the feeling we're experiencing in that moment is the most powerful part of the routine. Don't get me wrong: the calories we've burned are great, but the real money is the feeling we take away for the rest of our day. But no matter what I say in those final five minutes, the one thing I always do is ask them to "bottle up" that spirit we've tapped into so they can sprinkle that feeling throughout the rest of their day.

That's right. I ask them to take those extra few moments to close their eyes and recognize how their spirit feels right then. I ask them to have that moment with themselves when they can dial into the energy they've created from their workout that's enhancing not just their body but their mind and spirit as well. I get them to truly connect with how important that moment is to their day and their life.

Then, once they can connect to that energy, I ask them to transfer that spirit from the room into a bottle in their mind, seal it tight, then take it with them so they can take a sip of it whenever they need it most.

LIFT YOUR S.O.U.L.

In the next chapter, when I share with you how to put everything together into a single four-week program, you'll not only feel that same magic after every workout, but you'll also learn how to bottle up that feeling. But that doesn't mean you can't lift your spirit in other ways throughout the next twenty-eight days. In fact, I expect you to.

See, I believe it's important to not to wait for something external to make us happy. In the fitness world I see it all the time: people think that once they reach their goals—once they have the body they have always dreamt of or fit into the clothes they think will make them sexy—they will finally be happy. They assume their spirit will be flying high. But it doesn't always work that way.

When it comes to your spirit, you have to put the cart before the horse. Or in this case, put your spirit before your expectations. It's essential that you stimulate happiness from within because even though lifting your mind and body will make your spirit naturally rise as a result, the LIFTED program is about building awareness of all three simultaneously.

That's why over the next four weeks as you LIFT your mind through meditation and LIFT your body through exercise, you're also going to set yourself down a path of actively seeking out what will LIFT your spirit. You'll also be cutting loose the anchors—the things in place in your life right now, whether you're aware of them or not—that have been tying your spirit down all this time.

Each week I want you to try a variety of four to five things that each raise your spirit a little higher and, in some cases, higher than you could ever imagine.

Week 1: Seek it! These tricks and tactics are all based on actively looking for things that can elevate your spirit.

Week 2: Own It! The tips you'll be doing this week are all about new ways to look at things in your life right now to help your spirit grow.

Week 3: Understand it! This week all the strategies will help you understand your spirit just a little bit more so you magnify it!

Week 4: Lose it! In the final week it's all about removing the shackles that are holding your spirit down.

Just know this: I don't expect you to be able to do all of what I'm suggesting in each week or throughout the entire month. But even mastering just one out of all of them will LIFT your spirit way higher than it was at the very start. These are long-term tools—some of them you'll find you can use right away, and others may take some time. But they are always here for you to access and use.

With some of these tactics you may not be in the right mindset or spiritual place to take them on. For others it could be difficult even to wrap your head around what I'm asking you to do—for now. But don't worry: as you practice them, each becomes a lot easier.

But for now just do your best from week to week to at least *think* about each one, then attempt whichever tactics you think you can do. No matter which you choose to use, your spirit will thank you for it in the end.

The Three You'll Always Need

Even if you're not able to implement all the suggestions I'm going to ask you to try over the next four weeks, there are three things I need you to look for before you begin. Three important assets that as you follow the LIFTED program—and, for that matter, continue LIFTING yourself throughout your life—will always play critical roles in how far you're able to lift your spirit.

Find Out Where Your Spirit Lives

We all have one, and if you're lucky enough, you have several. That place that always seems to fill you with happiness. A place you turn to when you need to LIFT your spirits naturally.

Music can be a spirit-driven place, and it is for me. I'll show you how to get there next. But for now I want you to think of a physical place, one you'll never deny yourself having access to. Whatever place you choose, make sure you keep it local, as you may not have the freedom to pack your bags and travel someplace to LIFT your spirit over the next four weeks.

Maybe it's a special room in your house, a favorite restaurant, a certain spot in the library, or a particular path in the park you like to walk. It could be as simple as stepping outside no matter where you are and having sunshine on you. Wherever it may be, recognize it and be ready to visit it often along your journey. The more you do, the more you'll naturally raise your spirit without even trying.

Plan Your Own Spirit Soundtrack

I think one of the reasons my classes are so effective is that I spend so much time thinking of ways to wake up the spirit. I'll consider every single song played during each session and how each one will take my class on a journey.

When I do it, the songs I choose are based on what I need for that day. I may choose a song that I know will get me so excited that it makes me want to dance. The next song might make me a little introspective, reminding me of the struggles I've been through and have triumphed over. Or I might play a song that allows me to dig deep and reminds me that even though I have problems right now, I have always managed to overcome my challenges.

In the Body chapter I told you to create your own playlists for your workouts and even gave you some of my favorite recommendations. But why stop there?

Let's face it: we never know what life is going to throw at us outside of our workouts. Even if everything's going great today, we are aware we're going to have a few tomorrows that are going to be a little more challenging. Days when having something behind you to keep you going—a Spirit Soundtrack you can turn to and play in the background when your spirit doesn't want to fly—can be your greatest ally.

A lot of people understand the importance of a Spirit Soundtrack when you think about preparing for a long drive. When I get in my Jeep I've got the perfect Spirit Soundtrack for any trip. And when I play that music I want to make the experience even richer with the wind blowing through my hair and the sun on my face because it's almost like taking advantage of recharging my spirit the entire journey.

Thinking ahead and planning for those less-spirited days can make them a lot less stressful and a lot more joyous. So before they come, I want you to put serious thought into your music and prepare your own Spirit Soundtrack, one you can play in the background that will consciously and unconsciously lift you up on days when life is trying to pull you down.

My only tip: don't just throw in a bunch of upbeat songs. Spend the time to really think about where each song is going to take your spirit. Make it a collection of songs that doesn't just lift your spirit but also takes it someplace far away and out of reach from anything that might bring you down. That way, when you turn to it, it'll be that much more efficient at keeping your spirit where it should be—always up!

Find That Person Who Sees Your Gifts

Oftentimes we fail to see what's special about ourselves. We fail to recognize what gifts we bring to the world or what makes us unique. But there's always someone in our lives who sees us in a way we may not see ourselves.

When I feel like I don't know what makes me special or different, I get on the phone with my dad. He's been there from the very beginning and has watched my entire journey—he's even taken my spin classes and actually had tears in his eyes! I don't know how he does it, but he always has a way of saying things so perfectly.

Even if we sometimes don't believe what that person says, it always lifts the spirit when we touch base with those who recognize the positive things about us. The one who sees the gifts we don't allow ourselves to notice or may need a reminder that we have. So find yours, promise me you'll touch base with them often, and, most importantly, be willing to listen to the things they have to say about you.

LIFT . . . YOUR SPIRIT!

Week One: Seek It!

Carve Time for What Makes Your Heart Sing

Have you ever wondered why, in the event of an emergency on an airplane, the first thing you're instructed to do is put the oxygen mask on yourself? The answer is easy: if you don't take care of yourself first, you may not be able to take care of those around you.

It doesn't seem selfish when you fly, does it? Yet when it comes to helping your spirit soar, taking care of ourselves always seems to be last on our list. That's why I want you to write down a list of things that make you happy, then prioritize your day to make sure at least one of those things make their way into it. Make sure you're doing something each day that's guaranteed to make you smile.

Preferably, you should pencil them in for the morning so that whatever you choose isn't left for the end of the day when you may not have time to do them. If you can't do mornings, then schedule them like you would schedule anything in your life that is important to do. So if what you really need to make you happy is to be outside for a while, then schedule that time outdoors for a particular time of the day as if your job depended on it.

However, don't think of it as being selfish. After all, the same rules that you have no problem with up in the air apply down here on the ground as well. If you can't do something for your spirit, you're not going to be able to raise others' spirits.

Leave What's Familiar to Find Something New

A lot of times I get caught up in the same routine in the city. It's so easy to take the exact same route to the places I need to get to, and along the way, visit the same stores, walk the same streets, and see the same things I have seen while going from point A to point B that I had seeing from point B to point A.

But every once in a while, when I know my spirit needs it, I'll turn things on their head. It could be something as simple as just going down a different street or walking through an entirely different section of New York City entirely. It sounds small, but just that little shakeup in my life allows me to almost step outside of myself to see what else is out there and see things in a different way.

Sometimes I'll discover something I never knew existed. Other times I may see something that wakes up something from my past I had forgotten that I really enjoyed at one time. The fact is that our spirit can become grounded because there is too much routine in our lives. We forget to explore and get out as often as we should, when just taking a different path every so often can be like a tiny vacation that's enough to shake our spirit loose.

Find Something You Left Behind and Give It Wings

In class my classes I often say, "Today is my day. Now is my time. There are no obstacles in my way."

For a long time I thought that my time spent in basketball was my heyday. That was when I was going to do my best for my entire life. I felt so much that way that I genuinely believed that my greatest days were *then* and couldn't possibly be *right now*.

But I'm not alone. Many people carry that feeling in their spirit—the feeling that their best days are waaaaaay in the distance and so far behind them that there's no longer a need to try. That's why I also tell the people in my classes: "Depression is living in the past. Anxiety is living in the future. But happiness is all about being present."

Think about it: when you're anxious it's usually because you're worrying about something that may or may not happen. If you're depressed, it's usually about something you can't do anything about or do anymore. But your best days aren't behind you—they're right now. You could have an amazing tomorrow—it's just you holding yourself back today.

When I finally realized I was exactly where I needed to be at this moment in my life, that's when I begin to realize that my spirit was always capable of having its best day right now. So ask yourself: What did I leave behind that I always meant to do—and what's stopping me from doing it right now?

For me, it was surfing. There were so many things I didn't do when I played basketball because I didn't want to get hurt and the sport was paying the bills. Yet I always loved that surfer's mentality and the entire culture. So I tried it—at the age of thirty. And when I go in the water today some of the best surfers I see are in their forties and fifties. I could have let myself believe I was too old to try something new, but I knew I needed to keep myself in the mindset that it's never too late.

What's your forgotten thing?

Everybody has them—the things or moments they've left behind. I wouldn't expect you to find them all, but just choose one. It doesn't even have to be the most meaningful of them all, and you don't have to be perfect at it either. It's just important that you do it.

Just find one forgotten thing you know you can start moving on today so that you can experience that spirit-lifting sense of accomplishment after you eventually pull it off. So you have proof that just because you left a dream behind, it doesn't mean you can't ever go back to it years later and make it happen.

Help Somebody Every Day in Some Small Way

I'm so lucky to be an instructor where I get to help people. When others walk out of my class thanking me or saying things like, "You don't know what that did for me today!" it's almost unexplainable. I'm left so high from seeing the happiness on their faces and in their smiles, it elevates my spirit.

Every.

Single.

Time.

I teach about fifty people a class, fifteen times a week. If you do the math, you can imagine about how many little thank yous I get—little thank yous that build this reserve of energy in me that keeps my spirit perpetually afloat. And I understand that's something you might not be able to feel as often—but then again, what's stopping you? Today—and at least once every day moving forward—I want you to make a point of doing something nice for someone, preferably someone you don't even know.

It can sometimes be the smallest things that can have the biggest effect. Living in New York, I feel like I have the opportunity to do something kind all the time, as even just holding a door for a person is typically a startling surprise for a lot of people in NYC! But it doesn't have to be something so unusually unexpected as paying for coffee or the toll fare for the person behind you; it can be a gesture as little as smiling at someone or simply saying "Good morning!"—two things that take no time, effort, or extra cash at all.

You'll find plenty of those tiny moments waiting to LIFT your spirit throughout the day during those times when we find ourselves vying to beat the next guy. Those moments when your first instinct is usually to say, "Hey, it's my turn. This is all about me!"

If you pay attention to that instinct, whether it's rushing to beat someone to the checkout counter, jumping ahead of somebody to catch a cab, or trying to jockey for a great parking space, you'll find that moment. That chance to stop thinking about everything as being *your turn* and instead, stepping aside to allow it to be someone else's turn for a change.

When those moments happen, be honest with yourself about how much you're *really* going to lose in that moment. Most times, what does it really amount to? Waiting a little longer—or sometimes only a few seconds—more? Walking another forty feet because you had to park a few spaces over? It usually amounts to being just a few minutes late to something that probably isn't as important as you believe it is.

Yet by allowing somebody to come in first place and choosing second instead, you'll have done something that cost nothing for someone who didn't expect that act of kindness to come their way. An act of kindness that not only LIFTS your spirit because you know you've done something nice for someone but also just may LIFT their spirit in turn—or even better, inspired them to do the same thing to someone else during their day . . . yes, we really can pay it forward!

Find a New Way to Grow and Nurture It

We always tend to do the things we're good at rather than the things that challenge us. Why? Because it's easier and feels more comfortable to succeed at something we know how to do than struggling with something we don't.

But there's a whole lot of sense of accomplishment that comes from stepping outside our comfort zone and making ourselves vulnerable through trying something we may not be good at. It may not always be easy, and it might not be fun at first, but the reward is always greater when you're doing something that doesn't feel as comfortable.

A few years ago I took a hip-hop class but then stopped going because I wasn't that great at it. So I would text my friends to tell them I wasn't going that night. But then they would remind me how, when I did it, I was so excited and happy. They reminded me that I had made new friends and how the class broke down some walls inside of me.

I didn't see it at first because I couldn't look past feeling awkward, but the reward was worth not being the world's best hip-hop dancer.

After a certain point many of us stop growing not because we run out of ways to improve ourselves but because we stop putting ourselves in situations that give us the opportunity to learn something new. But the more you learn about things you didn't know before, the more you grow and begin to understand things about yourself right now.

So ask yourself: *What can I add to what I already am? What can I bring to myself that will make everything I am even better?* Make a short list, then find the one that makes you step out of your comfort zone the furthest—and jump right in.

Week Two: Own It!

Be Aware of What You Should Appreciate

A lot of times we become so focused on reaching for the next thing in our lives that we forget to take the time to look and see all the wondrous things we've already pulled within our grasp. We become too busy reaching to notice what we've already embraced, such as our health, good friends, certain accomplishments, or a steady job that we love.

There was a time when my life in basketball was always about reaching for the next thing. It was about perfecting my crossover. Then it was about getting my free-throw percentage up. Then it was about my need to be the leading scorer. And so on. And so on. And so on.

Striving for all those things and the many others that came before, in between, and after was great because it kept me driven and kept me succeeding. But many times I became so focused on striving that I forgot that I was already a top athlete. I just kept reaching instead of taking the time to appreciate things in the moment. That's why it's so important to recognize what we should be thankful for.

When you're thankful, it exposes your spirit to an abundance of positive things and improves your life in so many ways.

- It increases your happiness, which can lead to heightened well-being, which can bring you happiness that lasts. In a landmark study researchers found that subjects who took time to write and deliver a thank-you letter to someone they never properly thanked immediately felt a huge increase in happiness that lasted up to a month.[1]
- It can keep you healthy and fit. Research has shown that when people write down a few sentences about things they are grateful for each week, they not only feel more optimistic about their lives but also experience fewer visits to the doctor and tend to exercise more often.[2]
- It improves your sense of self-worth. A study published in the *Journal of Applied Sport Psychology* found that athletes who were grateful for their coaches experienced a noticeable boost in their self-esteem over time.[3]

- Your gratitude can make others feel grateful and, as a result, indirectly improve their lives as well. Research has shown mutual gratitude that leads to better and healthier relationships, as you'll feel more connected to people when you're grateful for each other.[4]
- According to science, gratitude improves your sleep quality and duration.[5] Meaning, if you count your blessings, you'll never count sheep!
- Finally, it reduces the desire for materialism.[6] The more you're grateful for, the less you'll find you need to acquire to be truly happy.

That's why starting this week I want you to write in a Gratitude Journal. That may sound like a lot of work, but I promise you that it's super easy. All I want you to do is write down three to five things you're grateful for right now.

However, I don't think you can ever be too grateful for too many things. So if you really want to write down another one or two, please—have at it! But just promise me you'll be careful. I want anything that's on that list to be genuine and heartfelt; if you put down too much, you might find yourself just going through the motions and writing just for the sake of writing. That's just not going to help you a whole lot.

Beyond that, there are no hard and fast rules as to how you do it. Everyone is grateful for different reasons—and your reasons will be as unique as you are—so just write the first few things that come to your mind. But I would recommend that you don't make them materialistic; instead, try to remember that you should be thankful for the most basic things in life. Maybe today you're just thankful that you're healthy because last week you were sick. At this point you're already seven days into the LIFTED program, so maybe you're grateful you made it through week one. Our families, our jobs, even something as simple as sunshine or the comfort of home—there is always plenty to be grateful for if you just take a moment to think about it.

Personally, I find the best day to write in my Gratitude Journal is a Sunday. That's the day most people plan the rest of their week out, and it's also the day most of us have fewer things going on, so there's less to distract you from digging deep and thinking about what you're thankful for.

Finally, once you've written your list, put it someplace where it can remind you of what you should be thankful for throughout your day. If that's in your bag, carry it everywhere you go. Or put it on a Post-it note and stick it on your desk so you have it to turn to every so often. But if having that list out there for anyone else to see might embarrass you, here's a trick: just place a sticker somewhere that will always remind you of what you wrote on Sunday. Whatever works for you is great so long as what you've written is always top of your mind rather than tucked away in a drawer.

Embrace Your Next Mistake—And Learn from It

No one's perfect, least of all me. And somewhere along the next four weeks you're going to make mistakes. It might be in the workout program or when you meditate, or it might be related to something entirely outside of LIFTED. Maybe you're not so great in a relationship with someone or not performing up to speed at your job. But you *will* stumble at some point because—that's right—mistakes happen.

As an athlete, I really had to learn the difference between being emotional and being passionate whenever I would make a mistake. Sometimes I would lose it and be upset with myself, but the only thing being mad at myself did was take me out of the game longer. I realized quickly that whenever I dwelled on my mistakes, it always held me back.

But when I spend time reflecting on *why* I was messing up in a game and then used that know-how to work on whatever skill I kept screwing up in order to prevent it from happening as often, not only did that help me move on but it also changed who I was at that moment.

Mistakes are an opportunity for us to have a little insight into ourselves. It's the best time to ask ourselves, Why did I stumble right there? and What can I do to prevent that from happening again—right now!

So when that next mistake comes—and it will—I don't want you to get angry or feel sorry for yourself, or worse, not accept the blame. Take a step back and try to *own* that mistake. Remind yourself that it's not the end of the world, figure out the trigger that caused it, then look for a way to remove it.

Cherish the Smallest of Victories

It's really important to have big goals and big dreams. But I also believe the only way you can accomplish big dreams is through tiny dreams. There is so much satisfaction in the smallest of victories, and if you could rewind your entire life, you would see how many small accomplishments made you happy along the way.

I dialed into this early in my life. When I was a kid I used to do a skills program designed by former player and basketball coach Steve Alford. It was a routine that had me perform and keep track of twenty-plus different moves all at once, and I had charts all over my garage. (In fact, I still have one of them!)

Thanks to these charts, I had percentages so I could track my progress little by little. I was able to recognize each accomplishment and feel successful right away and each and every day. And within two months I ended up being a better player. But to think I would've become a better player without having to build every little step of the way—to not have all these small accomplishments add up—would've been entirely unrealistic.

It's important to remember that your mind, body, and spirit are no different. As you experience the LIFTED program you're going to soar at a different speed from someone else trying the program alongside you—because we're all different. But as you go, I don't want you measuring anyone else but yourself. With each little tiny accomplishment—whether it's meditating five seconds longer than you did the last time, noticing a bit more of your abs peeking out, or doing something for your spirit you hadn't tried before—celebrate every single victory with the same amount of enthusiasm you'll show when you eventually reach and accomplish your dreams.

Peek Behind Your Passion

I used to think that basketball taught me to be a leader and allowed me to be a leader to other people. In actuality, however, I was always a leader. I would've wanted to guide others—as I do in my classes today—no matter what I did in life. That is who I am, and once I finally *owned* who I was rather than letting external things label me or dictate who I was, I found joy.

A lot of times we assume that the final destination is our passion. Maybe for you, it's earning a particular position at your job or visiting a place in the world where you've always wanted to travel. It's that thing we want to be or experience more than anything else. We all have a passion, but it's important to step back and ask yourself why that *thing* is so important to you.

If seeing the scale twenty pounds lighter is your goal, you need to ask yourself *why*. Is it because you like seeing that number, or do you think that number represents a different you? Someone who looks better and feels better? Is that what you want, or is there another reason why you think losing weight will make you happier?

If you don't ask yourself the real reasons why you're so passionate about achieving a certain goal, then when you finally reach it, it can sometimes leave you feeling unfulfilled. Peeking *behind* your passion to *really* get to the heart of why you want that goal so bad in the first place—and why you think it will make your spirit soar—may help you realize other ways you can LIFT your spirit as well. Or it might make you realize that your goal isn't that thing after all. Regardless of the outcome, just look at your dream with a magnifying glass to make sure that what you're dreaming about will genuinely make you happy when it comes true.

Search Your Heart for Someone to Forgive

Just imagine you were still upset about all the little things that bothered you throughout your entire lifetime. Not only would it be ridiculous, but it would be a huge waste of time, right? In fact, if I asked you to list *every single thing* that bothered you ten years ago, five years ago—even just last year!—I'll bet you would have a hard time remembering every single thing because you probably moved on from most of them. And that's good! Because if you could list all of them, you're probably not over them in the first place.

We have only a finite amount of energy to give toward our day, our goals, and ourselves, yet think about the amount of energy it takes to continuously be mad. When you harbor ill will toward someone—when you rehash the same issues you have with someone over and over again in your heart—you end up directing some of that energy toward that person, and it slows down your spirit.

When you think about it that way, what good does it ever do for you to hold on to your grievances? Wouldn't you rather free up that space? One of my Holly-isms is "Every end is a new beginning." So why wouldn't you want to forgive someone or something, knowing that by doing so, a new beginning for yourself starts immediately? Doesn't it just make more sense to free up that energy and put it toward the people you love and whatever goals you want to accomplish?

That said, I would never *expect* you to forgive everybody in your life. I'm looking for you to boost your spirit, not enter yourself into sainthood! But I want you to find one thing or one person you can forgive this week so you have someone or something that's no longer stealing energy from your spirit.

Week Three: Understand It!

Recognize Bad Vibes for What They Are

If you've ever felt rejected, you know it hurts. But did you know that when you experience rejection, the same neural pathways that get tripped when you experience physical pain are activated?[7] That's right. The same parts of your brain that light up on a brain scan when you're physically hurt light up when you get rejected by your boss, a player on the court, or someone you love.

One of my most powerful memories of rejection was when I was a girl in Lincoln, Nebraska, and I had just started playing basketball. I was practicing with someone who lived across the street, and he told me I couldn't play basketball because I was too short and that I should try another sport.

I can still recall that moment so clearly. I remember how the sky looked that day, what I was wearing, and exactly how old I was. And I'll never forget those words coming out of his mouth. But instead of absorbing that rejection—and believing his words in a way that kept my spirit down—I just remember looking at him and thinking to myself, *You don't know me. How could you possibly say what's ahead of me in my life?*

And from that point on, I turned that moment into fuel for my future.

Today I'm super-thankful for that moment and can honestly say it was that comment—those words of rejection—that became a driving force throughout my life. It was also the day I realized that just because somebody says you can't do something, it never means you can't do it.

Think about the last time someone rejected you. Yeah, this can be tough. But here's the key part of the exercise: remember, who is somebody else to tell you that you can't do something or that you're not good enough? I believe that most times rejection is really about the other person and not really about you. That might sound clichéd, but I believe that 99.9 percent of the time, that's the case.

If you honestly take yourself out of that initial entanglement of emotions, you'll find that people are usually in their own worlds, doing the things that serve themselves—and their words are really never about you. So think about that: think about the last person who rejected you—or even the one who hurt you the worst—and say to yourself, *You don't know me. How could you possibly say what's ahead of me in my life?* Use the feeling this gives you to fuel your future.

Let Mad Mellow for Twenty Breaths

When I was playing basketball in France and had the worst game ever—I mean, I didn't make a single shot!—at the end of the game I was so frustrated that I took the ball—and I drop kicked it into the stands.

Yeah. That was me.

I remember the second the ball went off my foot, I started thinking almost in slow motion: *Ohhhhhhhhh noooooooooo!* My response had been so immediate. I looked back at my coach, and for the rest of my life I will never forget the look of disbelief on her face. That one moment of letting my emotions take over in the wrong way had almost cost me my job and my entire contract in France.

And for what? For a game where I just didn't score any points? For one hour when I couldn't figure out a way to win, no matter how hard I tried? But instead of going back to the bench and having my teammates be there for me, I didn't let my mad mellow and almost lost everything I had worked toward since I was six.

When your spirit falls in certain moments, the reaction you have can quickly create a situation that could bring it down even further if you're not careful. Any wrong reaction could set off a chain reaction, turning small annoyances into major issues just by giving them more time or attention than they deserve. You know what I'm talking about: that text you probably shouldn't have sent, that comment you knew was a knee-jerk reaction—we've all been there.

One of the running themes of LIFTED that connects the mind, body, and spirit together falls back to your breath. At any given point your breath is going to either help you or hurt you. If I get myself into a huff and am so angry that I can feel my breath quickening, I'm going to have a much different reaction compared to when I take a few deep breaths and almost take a step outside myself to view the situation as if I'm an observer. (The meditation you practice as part of this program will help you get even better at this.)

There is so much wisdom in the simple act of counting to ten, but I think the longer you breathe, the more you can prevent a flicker from turning into a fire. So from this point forward, when something upsets your spirit, I want you to take not ten but twenty deep breaths as slowly as possible and count each inhale and exhale. Look at it as spirit insurance. You'll immediately feel yourself physically calm down, and even though your spirit might still be low temporarily, you'll be preventing yourself from making the wrong choices that could keep it lower even longer.

Be Your Own Best Friend

We're so good at looking in the mirror and seeing what's wrong with ourselves, aren't we? Most people are pretty amazing at pointing out when they've missed a workout or screwed up on their diet. But what we're kind of really bad at is being supportive for ourselves and saying, "Hey! Good job . . . me!"

I don't know why it's so hard for us to be there for ourselves, especially when most of us are so good at being there for others. When someone succeeds in life our initial instinct is to tell them how happy that makes us—and it makes them happy too.

Any time a client comes up to me and says, "Holly! I ate great last week!" or "I meditated twice yesterday!" I tell them "I'm so proud of you!" And it lifts my spirit because I truly am. But how often do we give ourselves that pat on the back? How good would that feel to look in the mirror and for once say to yourself, "I love my legs!" or just think about something you admire about yourself.

Although it's hard for many people to practice self-compassion and not be judgmental toward themselves, it's necessary to love oneself—wrinkles and all. When we become our biggest cheerleader, when we talk to ourselves in the same way we would talk to a friend, we make ourselves less susceptible to failure, anxiety, stress, and rejection. We prevent ourselves from holding down our spirit and instead, give our spirit something to grow from.

So this week—starting today and every day after—I want you to look in the mirror and recognize the best friend you never knew you had.

Listen to Those Who Love You

When I first came to NYC in 2007, it wasn't to help shape the minds, bodies, and spirits of others through my classes. No, believe it or not, after I stopped playing professional ball, the fire that was once inside me—the one that basketball always kept lit—was gone. (Or so I thought.) So I stepped away from the world of fitness for a while and was determined to make it in real estate.

Back then I was so scared of the city that I would run down the West Side Highway with my sunglasses on to hide my tears. I thought to myself, *How can I possibly find my way here? And will I ever find that fire inside myself again?*

Then a friend of mine came up from Atlanta to stay with me. I had just moved into a one-bedroom apartment I couldn't afford, and all I had was a mattress in the middle of the living room. Hearing that, she told me we were going to do some "street shopping." And that's exactly what we did. We found a dresser, this old school desk, and a few other things on the street that made an empty room finally seem like home.

But it wasn't just having a familiar face around that was so nice—it was the fact that she cared so much that she took a risk by telling me to listen to something I wasn't hearing in myself. She looked at me and said, "What are you doing? You have a gift—and it's not in real estate. You belong in fitness, and I wish you would just wake up and realize that."

I could hear her saying the words, and I felt them resonate somewhere inside me, but I still was so disconnected from that place within my spirit that was willing to take a chance. I didn't think that the fire that had burned inside for decades for basketball would ever show up again. But eventually I knew she was right.

The fact is that sometimes our paths aren't so clear. But when friends, family, teachers, coaches, or someone you know who cares about you has the courage to step up and tell you you're getting in your own way, then you're being given a gift again—so listen to it.

This week keep your ears open to the lessons we sometimes need to learn from others. Right now there may be someone trying to tell you something. It might be something you're not ready to hear or something you continue to hear but aren't ready to listen to. If that person's out there, give them your time, give them your ear, and give them your love for thinking enough about you to recognize what may help your spirit grow.

Week Four: Lose It!

Don't Dread—Dream Instead

When Jillian Michaels left the *Biggest Loser*, I was up to replace her not once—but twice. Not getting the opportunity two times in a row crushed me, and there were times when I wondered how I ever could go back and teach again. After all, I had planned the rest of my life around being NBC's number-one trainer.

But just then someone told me to "trust the process."

Trusting the process not only allowed another television show to come along for me with Bravo; it also made those tough moments easier because I realized it's not just about that particular moment—it's about all moments combined. All of your moments eventually lead somewhere, and none of your drive, passion, and determination is ever wasted just because you didn't reach a dream.

When you trust the process, you can't just trust parts of it—you need to trust all of it. And when you do, life has a funny way of making things happen for you when you need it to.

Since learning to trust the process, I look around at things happening in my life at the moment that may not be ideal but also may not be as bad as they seem. For example, sometimes when I'm sick, instead of being upset about it or trying to push myself harder than I should be pushing, I'll actually say to myself, "I need this! My body needs a break."

I now look at those moments when life is slowing me down or stopping me from doing something through a different lens. In other words, instead of dreading the moment, I've come to realize that it's sometimes better to accept a situation that's out of your control, then think about how you could better yourself in the meantime.

For example, one critical time when life threw me a curveball was when I had a snowboarding injury just a few years ago. The accident left me with spinal compression, and I couldn't walk without pain for about a week. I couldn't teach spin classes, and even worse, I couldn't lift weights for about six months.

I was terrified.

The truth of the matter was that I hadn't taken a break from lifting for almost twenty years straight. Those six months would be the first time I hadn't done any weight training since I was in my twenties. But instead of dreading those six months, I was determined to make the best of them. So during that time I focused on my diet and experimented with other types of exercises that I was allowed to do. And soon my body was the best it had ever been in over a decade!

Who knew there could be a silver lining when I had a snowboarding accident—but there was one. But if I hadn't had that mentality, if I just had let everything go to hell

If You're Afraid to Fail . . . Read This!

You might be intimidated by some of the things—if not all—I'm asking you to do for your mind, body, and spirit. If that's you, then let me tell you a little story, an event that not only changed my life but also how I approach fitness to this day.

It was a while back when I first heard about this amazing yoga instructor in New York City named Dana Flynn, founder of Laughing Lotus Yoga Center and renowned for her levitating yoga classes. I knew I wanted to experience her class for myself, but I was intimated.

How was that possible? Here I was, a former professional athlete, but yoga? That was a completely different world for me!

When I walked into her class it was mat to mat—not a single additional body could squeeze itself into that room if they tried. I could actually feel the breath of the person behind me because they were so close! I was instantly intimidated, nervous, and super-self-conscious, and there was no turning back.

Once the class began, my focus went everywhere *but* inward. Instead, I was too busy looking at the people next to me to make sure my leg was in the right place and my arm wasn't bent in the wrong direction. I felt so outside myself, whereas everybody else in the class was very much in their own vibe, moving so fluidly and effortlessly. About halfway through I felt defeated, self-conscious, and embarrassed. I was such a hot mess that at one point I just sat on my mat and looked around and honestly thought I was ruining the class.

When it was all over I walked up to the instructor and told her how deeply sorry I was that I was a distraction in her class. And with that, she turned to look at me and said without missing a beat, "Oh, honey! No one was looking at you."

It was simple and to the point. It was painfully obvious. And at that moment it was true. Everything's not about me! No one was focusing on my mistakes. They were focusing on themselves and, more than likely, experiencing their own imperfections.

Those eight little words had such a profound effect on me, and it became a pivotal moment in my life. It was the day I came to truly understand that as much as we might think otherwise, people really aren't paying attention to us as much as we think they are. It's just our own little insecurities that make us believe that everybody is looking at us and scrutinizing everything we do.

It's those silly little misconceptions that many times are really holding us back.

The thing to remember is that this program is for life. It's truly not what happens to us along the way but how we handle it. Just remember that you don't have to be perfect—you just need to be willing. This day—and every day after—will be what you make it. So choose to shine!

and spent the entire time being upset, eaten poorly, and stayed in a bad mood, there wouldn't have been a silver lining.

This week look for that situation that's leaving you feeling unlucky, then figure out a way to turn that negative thing into something positive. And if there's nothing going on with you, that's fantastic! But from this day forward just remember that the next time you're faced with a situation that makes you normally think, *Why me?* try to figure out a way to turn it into an opportunity to say, "Lucky me!"

Misery Loves Company—So Let It Fly Solo

Sometimes when we feel sad and depressed, we tend to gravitate toward music, movies, books, TV shows, or other forms of entertainment that are in line with how we feel. That's because for many of us there's some weird sense of comfort reading about, watching, or listening to something in sync with how miserable we feel. Maybe it makes us feel less alone at that moment, but what it sometimes can do is root us longer in an emotion that's keeping our spirit down.

The problem is that when you align yourself with misery, it keeps you in that emotion. It makes you a little more likely to stay sadder longer because you're never letting yourself naturally become happier. You're keeping yourself depressed by surrounding yourself with things that are depressing. Misery loves company? Misery loves misery!

I think it's important to understand that at any second and any moment—night or day—you have a choice. There's never this big weight that you can't get off your chest. No, you have a choice: you can choose from a variety of options, and every choice leads to a slightly different feeling in a slightly different moment. So when misery comes knocking, don't join it; instead, shy away from anything depressing, like a sad movie, somber music, or a tragic novel. Know that those things may do more harm than good.

The same thing goes for toxic people in your life. I have my own struggles with things, and you know what? I also have a great set of people and friends around me. But I can tell you this much: over the last five years, with the success I've had, there are also people in my life that I have to be careful about connecting with because of jealousy or competition.

Remember the analogy of putting on your own oxygen mask first? Well, it also works in reverse. If you have a friend who is sucking the oxygen out of you, you're both going to go down.

By now you're more in tune with your spirit after using the LIFTED program for over three weeks. And because of that, you're going to know when you're around people who are holding your spirit back. I've become so in tune with it that there are certain people I know suck the spirit out of me—and I can feel it happening immediately. Those are people I've had to cut out at all costs, and I encourage you to do the same.

But I get it. When you're a good person with a good heart, it's hard to turn your back on a friend, even if that friend may be pulling you down. That friend who says, every time you talk to her, that the world is always against her. That friend who is always miserable instead of thankful or happy. That friend who, because you're a good person, you may feel compelled to stay with, even though you've never been able to turn her around.

Just remember that you're never held hostage to anything and that you always have a choice. Then tell that friend about the steps you're taking and how it's improving your life. Make sure she knows that *I'm only telling you this because I need to take care of myself first, and I care about you, but I'm going to make these changes.*

You need to understand that you need to be responsible for your own happiness. And then, hopefully, you will lead by example and show that friend the way you could never convince her was possible.

Take Away a Plate or Two

Maybe you're the type who likes to tell people how many plates you're spinning because you're proud to be a multitasker—and I get that! There's a rush to being able to keep a thousand and one plates in the air. But if you're not careful, saying that you'll do something then not delivering on that promise can also make you feel like a failure or lower someone's opinion of you. Either way, the result torpedoes your spirit, even though you had the best of intentions.

It's not always your fault. Sometimes life honestly gets in the way and prevents us from getting something done. But other times it might be because we wrote a check that our ass just couldn't cash.

When you take too much on, you set yourself up to possibly fail. And when you fail, you may beat yourself up to the point where it brings down your spirit. It's a vicious circle, but here's the thing: we often have control over it because it's just a matter of prioritizing better. All it takes is being careful not to overwhelm ourselves, either because we feel we need to or because we have something to prove.

So this week I want you to find one of your spinning plates and take it down—for now. And with the rest I want you to follow through, and from this point on, never bite off more than you can chew.

Besides lessening the stress that comes from trying to juggle too many things at once, there's a real spirit-lifting boost we get whenever we check something off our list. Better yet, once you follow through with something and get it done, it will instantly make you realize what other things you could be accomplishing if you gave yourself a break and lightened your load.

Expect Nothing in Return

The final tip I have for you is, lose the expectation of appreciation. What do I mean by that? This chapter is filled with things to try that can make you a better person, and each goes a long way in LIFTING your spirit. That's what I want you to remember most of all—that you've tried some (or all) of these for *you* and not for someone else.

By taking on some of these spirit-LIFTING challenges, you'll be doing nice things for other people. But the one thing I don't want you to do is to expect that same sense of spirit in return.

When you do something nice for somebody, it doesn't always have to come with a thank you. It doesn't always end with a smile. You're almost waiting for that endorphin rush to be released, and if it doesn't come, it's easy to feel this empty place. Maybe that's the reason you stopped doing some of these things along the way. Maybe when you tried, it never felt like you were making a difference or that every time you helped someone it indirectly hurt you in return in a small way because you were never thanked or appreciated.

But this book is about LIFTING yourself up so you can be better for other people—and for yourself. The truth of the matter is that regardless of whether or not you get thanked, you've done something to help yourself. You've done something to make yourself happier and a better person. Looking for someone to acknowledge your niceness almost cheapens it in a way when you think about it. After all, you should never do something nice for the thank you and the smile—those are just the bonuses that sometimes come along the way.

Follow these guidelines for your spirit—and never for the praise. Now get going.

5

Bring It All Together:
The LIFTED Program—In a Nutshell

Now that you know what to do for your mind, your body, and your spirit, you have two options to choose from to bring it all together into one program: an "express" version, which is based on shorter workouts that LIFT the mind, body, and spirit, or hour-long workout sessions designed in the same way as my classes. If you're looking for a LIFTED experience that's as close as possible to what I do with my class, then the longer version is for you.

The Guidelines

No matter which version you try, the rules are simple:

- Follow the LIFTED program for four weeks straight.
- Do what is required in all three sections: mind, body, and spirit. (I don't want you doing only two sections, and I definitely don't want you doing only one. It's all three or nothing.)
- Each week make the required changes to the program within all three sections so you LIFT yourself even further.
  So you have them all in one place, now here are the changes you should make each week:

Week One

MIND

Meditate for a minimum of ten minutes every day for seven days. (You'll also meditate as described within each workout.)

BODY

Just follow the workout program described in Chapter 5, including Dynamic Warm-Up and Cool-Down Stretches.

SPIRIT

Complete at least one of the Seek It! goals. Even if you think you can't, I know you can do at least one. If you can do more, I'm proud of you!

DAY 1 UPPER BODY	DAY 2 LOWER BODY	DAY 3 ABS
10 Push Ups	10 Glute Bridges	10 Bird Dogs
Side Plank (right side only) [30 seconds]	10 Squats	Plank [30 seconds]
10 Dips	Plank [30 seconds]	High Knees [30 seconds]
Mountain Climbers [30 seconds]	20 Reverse Lunges [10 reps each leg]	Russian Twists [30 seconds]
Side Plank (left side only) [30 seconds]	2 Wall Sits [30 seconds]	High Knees [30 seconds]
10 Renegade Rows [5 each arm]	10 Single-Leg Romanian Deadlifts (balance on right leg)	10 Reach Backs [5 each side]
High Knees [30 seconds]	High Knees [30 seconds]	4 Rockstars [2 each side]
10 Up-Down Planks	10 Up-Down Planks	10 Goddess Sit Ups
Fast Feet [30 seconds]	Fast Feet [30 seconds]	Fast Feet [30 seconds]
		10 V-ups
		High Plank with Shoulder Taps [do for 30 seconds]
		10 Burpees

Rest for 60 seconds,
then start at the beginning

DAY 4 CARDIO DAY	DAY 5 UPPER BODY	DAY 6 LOWER BODY	DAY 7 OFF
Do 30 minutes' worth of sprint intervals (sprint for 30 seconds, then recover for 60 seconds by either walking or putting your hands over your head to refocus so you can go hard again immediately. Repeat 20 times total.)	10 Push Ups Side Plank (right side only) [30 seconds] 10 Dips High Planks with Shoulder Taps [30 seconds] Mountain Climbers [30 seconds] 10 Up-Down Planks Sumo Squat Fighters [30 seconds] 10 Renegade Rows [5 each arm] Speed Skaters [30 seconds]	10 Glute Bridges 10 Single-Leg Romanian Deadlifts (balance on right leg) 10 Squats 10 Single-Leg Romanian Deadlifts (balance on left leg) Plank [30 seconds] 10 Plyo Lunges (right leg only) Side Plank (right side only) [30 seconds] 10 Plyo Lunges (left leg only) Side Plank (left side only) [30 seconds] 10 Drop Squats Fast Feet [30 seconds]	REST

Rest for 60 seconds,
then start at the beginning

Week Two

MIND

Add one minute more to your meditation session so you're meditating for a minimum of eleven minutes every day. (You'll also meditate as described within each workout.)

BODY

As I mentioned in Chapter 5, to make the workout more intense, you'll add either four additional repetitions or five more seconds of time to each exercise.

Continue to rest sixty seconds at the end of each circuit. Begin with the Dynamic Warm-Up and end with Cool-Down Stretches.

SPIRIT

Complete at least one of the Own It! goals. If you can do more, keep going! But if you can't, your spirit will still soar even if you only do just one.

DAY 1 UPPER BODY	DAY 2 LOWER BODY	DAY 3 ABS
12 Push Ups	12 Glute Bridges	12 Bird Dogs
Side Plank (right side only) [35 seconds]	12 Squats	Plank [35 seconds]
12 Dips	Plank [35 seconds]	High Knees [35 seconds]
Mountain Climbers [35 seconds]	22 Reverse Lunges [11 reps each leg]	Russian Twists [35 seconds]
Side Plank (left side only) [35 seconds]	Wall Sits [35 seconds]	High Knees [35 seconds]
12 Renegade Rows [6 each arm]	12 Single-Leg Romanian Deadlifts (balance on right leg)	12 Reach Backs [6 each side]
High Knees [35 seconds]	12 Single-Leg Romanian Deadlifts (balance on left leg)	6 Rockstars [3 each side]
12 Up-Down Planks	12 Burpees	12 Goddess Sit Ups
Fast Feet [35 seconds]		Fast Feet [35 seconds]
		12 V-ups
		High Plank with Shoulder Taps [do for 35 seconds]
		12 Burpees

Rest for 60 seconds, then start at the beginning

DAY 4 CARDIO DAY	DAY 5 UPPER BODY	DAY 6 LOWER BODY	DAY 7 OFF
Do 30 minutes' worth of sprint intervals (sprint for 30 seconds, then recover for 60 seconds by either walking or putting your hands over your head to refocus so you can go hard again immediately. Repeat 20 times total.)	12 Push Ups Side Plank (right side only) [35 seconds] 12 Burpees Side Plank (left side only) [35 seconds] 12 Dips High Planks with Shoulder Taps [35 seconds] Mountain Climbers [35 seconds] 12 Up-Down Planks Sumo Squat Fighters [35 seconds] 12 Renegade Rows [6 each arm] Speed Skaters [35 seconds]	12 Glute Bridges 12 Single-Leg Romanian Deadlifts (balance on right leg) 12 Squats 12 Single-Leg Romanian Deadlifts (balance on left leg) Plank [35 seconds] 12 Plyo Lunges (right leg only) Side Plank (right side only) [35 seconds] 12 Plyo Lunges (left leg only) Side Plank (left side only) [35 seconds] 12 Drop Squats Fast Feet [35 seconds]	REST

Rest for 60 seconds, then start at the beginning

Week Three

MIND

Add one minute more to your meditation session so you're meditating for a minimum of twelve minutes every day. (You'll also meditate as described within each workout.)

BODY

Add another four additional repetitions or five more seconds of time to each exercise. Lower the amount of time you'll rest at the end of each circuit to forty-five seconds instead of sixty. Begin with the Dynamic Warm-Up and end with Cool-Down Stretches.

SPIRIT

Complete at least one of the Understand It! goals. The more you do, the better you'll understand your spirit. But if you can only do one, you're still doing it!

DAY 1 UPPER BODY	DAY 2 LOWER BODY	DAY 3 ABS
14 Push Ups	14 Glute Bridges	14 Bird Dogs
Side Plank (right side only) [40 seconds]	14 Squats	Plank [40 seconds]
14 Dips	Plank [40 seconds]	High Knees [40 seconds]
Mountain Climbers [40 seconds]	24 Reverse Lunges [12 reps each leg]	Russian Twists [40 seconds]
Side Plank (left side only) [40 seconds]	Wall Sits [40 seconds]	High Knees [40 seconds]
14 Renegade Rows [7 each arm]	14 Single-Leg Romanian Deadlifts (balance on right leg)	14 Reach Backs [7 each side]
High Knees [40 seconds]	14 Single-Leg Romanian Deadlifts (balance on left leg)	8 Rockstars [4 each side]
14 Up-Down Planks	14 Burpees	14 Goddess Sit Ups
Fast Feet [40 seconds]		Fast Feet [40 seconds]
		14 V-ups
		High Plank with Shoulder Taps [do for 40 seconds]
		14 Burpees

Rest for 45 seconds, then start at the beginning

DAY 4 CARDIO DAY	DAY 5 UPPER BODY	DAY 6 LOWER BODY	DAY 7 OFF
Do 30 minutes' worth of sprint intervals (sprint for 30 seconds, then recover for 60 seconds by either walking or putting your hands over your head to refocus so you can go hard again immediately. Repeat 20 times total.)	14 Push Ups Side Plank (right side only) [40 seconds] 14 Burpees Side Plank (left side only) [40 seconds] 14 Dips High Planks with Shoulder Taps [40 seconds] Mountain Climbers [40 seconds] 14 Up-Down Planks Sumo Squat Fighters [40 seconds] 14 Renegade Rows [7 each arm] Speed Skaters [40 seconds]	14 Glute Bridges 14 Single-Leg Romanian Deadlifts (balance on right leg) 14 Squats 14 Single-Leg Romanian Deadlifts (balance on left leg) Plank [40 seconds] 14 Plyo Lunges (right leg only) Side Plank (right side only) [40 seconds] 14 Plyo Lunges (left leg only) Side Plank (left side only) [40 seconds] 14 Drop Squats Fast Feet [40 seconds]	REST

Rest for 45 seconds,
then start at the beginning

Week Four

MIND

In this final week add one minute more to your meditation session so you're meditating for a minimum of thirteen minutes every day. (You'll also meditate as described within each workout.)

BODY

Add another four additional repetitions or five more seconds of time to each exercise. Lower the amount of time you rest at the end of each circuit to thirty seconds instead of forty-five. Begin with the Dynamic Warm-Up and end with Cool-Down Stretches.

SPIRIT

Complete at least one of the Lose It! goals. If you can do more, your spirit will thank you for it! But if you can't, just doing one will free your spirit in such a way that when you try the program again, you'll be eager to do more.

DAY 1 UPPER BODY	DAY 2 LOWER BODY	DAY 3 ABS
16 Push Ups	16 Glute Bridges	16 Bird Dogs
Side Plank (right side only) [45 seconds]	16 Squats	Plank [45 seconds]
16 Dips	Plank [45 seconds]	High Knees [45 seconds]
Mountain Climbers [45 seconds]	20 Reverse Lunges [10 reps each leg]	Russian Twists [45 seconds]
Side Plank (left side only) [45 seconds]	Wall Sits [45 seconds]	High Knees [45 seconds]
16 Renegade Rows [8 each arm]	16 Single-Leg Romanian Deadlifts (balance on right leg)	16 Reach Backs [8 each side]
High Knees [45 seconds]	16 Single-Leg Romanian Deadlifts (balance on left leg)	10 Rock Stars [5 each side]
16 Up-Down Planks	16 Burpees	16 Goddess Sit Ups
Fast Feet [45 seconds]		Fast Feet [45 seconds]
		16 V-ups
		High Plank with Shoulder Taps [45 seconds]
		16 Burpees

Rest for 30 seconds, then start at the beginning

DAY 4 CARDIO DAY	DAY 5 UPPER BODY	DAY 6 LOWER BODY	DAY 7 OFF
Do 30 minutes of sprint intervals (sprint for 30 seconds, then recover for 60 seconds by either walking or putting your hands over your head to refocus so you can go hard again immediately. Repeat 20 times total.)	16 Push Ups Side Plank (right side only) [45 seconds] 16 Burpees Side Plank (left side only) [45 seconds] 16 Dips High Planks with Shoulder Taps [45 seconds] Mountain Climbers [45 seconds] 16 Up-Down Planks Sumo Squat Fighters [45 seconds] 16 Renegade Rows [8 each arm] Speed Skaters [45 seconds]	16 Glute Bridges 16 Single-Leg Romanian Deadlifts (balance on right leg) 16 Squats 16 Single-Leg Romanian Deadlifts (balance on left leg) Plank [45 seconds] 16 Plyo Lunges (right leg only) Side Plank (right side only) [45 seconds] 16 Plyo Lunges (left leg only) Side Plank (left side only) [45 seconds] 16 Drop Squats Fast Feet [45 seconds]	REST

Rest for 30 seconds, then start at the beginning

Which Way Will You LIFT Yourself Today?

I know how to push myself—and my job is to push you that hard. To do that, I've done my best to give you the tools to create what you would experience if you came to New York City and experienced one of my LIFTED classes in person.

Traditionally my class is a sixty-minute mind, body, and spirit experience that's a combination of meditation, exercise, and taking a moment to bask and bottle the spirit you've stirred up during your workout so you can access it later at any time.

Yes, it takes over an hour, and that might be more than you bargained for. But just like I tell my class: the more uncomfortable you get in here, the more comfortable you are out there. I work out because I love my body—not because I hate it—and now it's your turn to do the same. So if you're ready, close your eyes, and let everything outside whatever room you are training in just disappear. Because you and I, we're going to see how many times we can lose our breath today.

The Full LIFTED Workout

This fuller version incorporates two seated meditations, two varied-length bursts of high-intensity exercise, and a five-minute finale when you'll lie down and bottle up the spirit you've ignited during your workout.

- Start with five minutes of meditation.
- Do the Dynamic Warm-Up.
- Do the LIFTED workout. Repeat the circuit until twenty-eight minutes are up. If you reach twenty-eight minutes but haven't performed at least three circuits total, keep moving until you've run through the circuit three times.
- Perform five more minutes of meditation.
- Do the LIFTED workout circuit one final time. (Don't do it for a particular time in minutes—just run through the entire series of exercises once more.)
- Do the Cool-Down Stretches.
- Finally, Bottle It Up for five minutes!

For these last five minutes I want you to lie down, letting your arms fall by your sides. Close your eyes, and simply surrender to the moment. Just acknowledge what you've done, how what you've accomplished has made you feel, and then bottle up that feeling and save it for later. Remember the magic you've created, so at any time during the day, especially during times when you need it most, you can close your eyes and take a sip.

The "Less Time, Same LIFT" Version

Strength does not always roar; in fact, sometimes it's the quiet voice at the end of the day that says, "I'll try again tomorrow."

If your time is less than you expected any given day or you're a beginner who is looking to ease into the LIFTED program, this slightly shorter version works just as well for your mind, body, and spirit.

- Start with five minutes of meditation.
- Do the Dynamic Warm-Up.
- Do the LIFTED workout. (Repeat the circuit until twenty-eight minutes are up. If you reach twenty-eight minutes but haven't performed at least three circuits total, keep moving until you've run through the circuit three times.)
- Do the Cool-Down Stretches.
- Finally, Bottle It Up for five minutes!

Bottle It Up Bonus!

When I ask my class to bottle up their spirit, they aren't just lying on the ground quietly—they are listening to me guide them through the process. And although I can't be there in your living room, on the beach, or whatever amazing place you've chosen to LIFT your mind, body, and spirit, that's what I want to do for you.

If you go to my website (holly.life), you'll find a downloadable version of me talking to my class afterward—so you can experience it for yourself. But if that's not an option for you, I'd like to share the following few paragraphs. These are words from the heart that I say in class quite often. These are some of the inspirational phrases I use to help my classes capture all the magical energy they've created so they can tap into it anytime they like.

Here's what I want you to do: have a close friend or family member read the following few paragraphs into your phone; if you're comfortable hearing your own voice, you'll do just fine too. Then save it and play it each time you need to Bottle Up your spirit at the end of any workout.

"THIS is the reason we do this. This moment right here. THIS is the reason we push ourselves so hard. The calories we burn are nice. But it's this feeling right now—this is the reason we come back time and time again.

Feel your heart beating a little faster. Notice your chest rise and fall with your breath. Pay attention to how far away your day has been for the past hour. How connected you felt to yourself. Notice how empowered, courageous, and confident you feel right now, in this very moment. Close your eyes. Soak it in. Breathe it in. Take a snapshot of it. And Bottle It Up. So later today or tomorrow morning when you wake up, you can take a sip of it when you need it. Remember that this feeling is only a breath away. We are always closer to okay than we think. In fact, it's usually right there next to you."

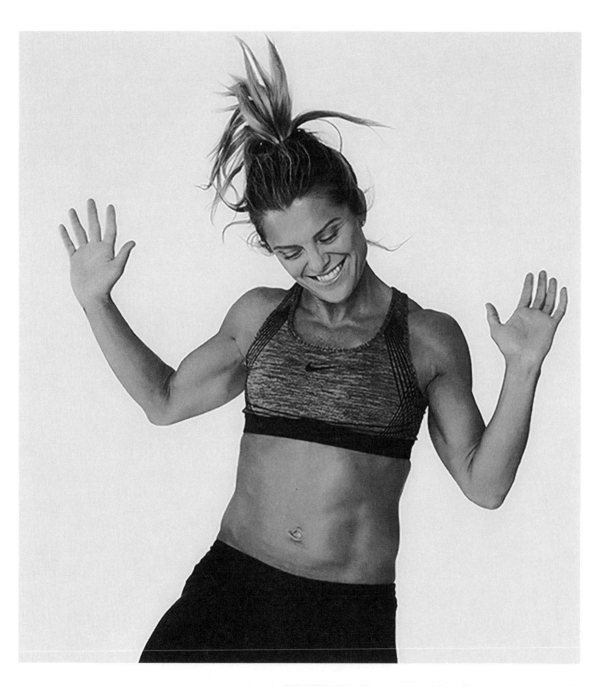

LIFTED FOR LIFE

6

Fuel Your Mind, Body, and Spirit!

First off, this isn't a diet book.

I would never be so bold as to think I could prescribe the exact number of times you should eat in a day because I don't know what's sustainable for you. I don't know about your life or if you have fifteen-hour work shifts that you're dealing with. I don't know if you have kids leaving half-finished plates you feel the need to eat so nothing goes to waste or if you have a chocolate habit you just can't kick.

I quite honestly don't know what you may need nutritionally. But the good news is that your mind, body, and spirit do—if you take the time to listen to them. So when it comes to what you should eat or drink, this chapter is filled with more "try-it" advice than diet advice. What I'm giving you are all the tools to help you drive your own life instead of having me drive it for you.

That doesn't mean what I'm about to teach you won't lead to losing body fat. By following the LIFTED program and raising your mind, body, and spirit simultaneously, you're going to naturally find yourself reaching less for certain comfort foods because you'll find comfort from within yourself—and not from a bunch of unhealthy eats.

The LIFTED Nutritional Lifestyle

If you're waiting for me to say, "Eat three meals and two snacks," or "Eat five small meals throughout the day," you'll be waiting a long time. Even though you may be used to seeing super-strict eating plans, you won't find one here because I feel that if any program requires too much of somebody, it becomes so daunting that you're less likely to do it.

Don't get me wrong: I think that being super-strict has its place. In fact, I believe that sometimes we need a little kick in the pants when we're not able to live a balanced life. That's not just with nutrition, but a lot of different areas in life. But I also think that when you look over the years of your life—I mean really look at the "big picture"—it's in those moments when you're highly restrictive, when you tell yourself you can't have things or you're too harsh about pulling everything out of your diet, that you end up stripping out a lot of the joy in your life.

Personally, I don't follow a set eating program, and when I see routines that spell out exactly what to eat every single day for every single meal, that's not for me. Instead, I feel it's important to give more leeway and simpler choices rather than being too strict. There are certain days when I don't eat a snack and my lunch takes me right into dinner. There are other days, especially after I've had a hard workout in the morning, when I'm starving every hour on the hour. All I do is listen to my body and remind myself of the difference between eating because I'm hungry and just looking to eat.

No, I'm not going to tell you when to eat along your four-week LIFTED journey because we already have this amazing internal mechanism called hunger. With so many diets and programs out there focused on what you should eat and how much you should eat, there's something to be said about dialing things back a bit, going back to the basics, and just asking yourself, Do I really need to eat, or am I eating for another reason?

Maybe that advice is too open-ended for you, but by just being mindful, it becomes much easier to figure out when you should eat and when you don't need to. It is about listening to your body, then asking yourself why you're about to eat what's about to go into your mouth—it's really that simple. That's why I'm a big believer in having a Food Journal—and so is science! In fact, a landmark study out of the Fred Hutchinson Cancer Research Center found that women who kept a food journal consistently lost an average of around six pounds more than women who didn't.[1]

My rules are easy:

1. Record everything you eat, but start by writing down the time of day.
2. Jot down the approximate portion size of each food. I'm totally against counting grams unless that's something you like to do. So if you can say "palm size" or "small piece," that's fine.
3. If a food was prepared, then remind yourself how, such as baked, fried, broiled, marinated, coated in dressing, and so forth.
4. Finally, if you want to dig deeper, ask yourself why you ate what you did—and whether there were feelings attached to that food. This might be especially helpful if you find yourself going to the fridge when it's not mealtime.

What do I mean by that? Simple: when it comes to every single food you write down, ask yourself the following questions in the exact order given:

- Did I eat this to be *social*? (If so, put a capital S next to it.)
- Did I eat this out of *tradition* and routine? (If so, put a capital T next to it.)
- Did I eat this out of *impulse* because of something emotional? (If so, put a capital I next to it.)
- Did I eat this out of *boredom*? (If so, put a capital B next to it.)
- Did I eat this to *avoid* something? (If so, put a capital A next to it.)
- Finally, ask yourself: Did I eat this because I was genuinely *hungry*? (If so, put a capital H next to it.)

The most impressive Food Journal should be filled with nothing but H's—and not because it's the first letter in my name. Unfortunately, often what we eat is attached to something that's happening in that moment of our lives. You may be eating because of the activity you're about to do or because you have absolutely nothing to do. You may be eating because everyone around you is or you're using food as a way to avoid dealing with someone or something, or because you feel like crap about something.

I do this a lot when I get an email I don't want to deal with. Because my office is right next to my kitchen, I'll find myself getting up to see what's in my refrigerator only because I'm trying to delay answering that email. But I know the difference between standing at my fridge to avoid stress versus being hungry, so when I have to come back to my Food Journal and write down a big "A" next to whatever bad food I just threw back, it hurts.

And that's good—because I like that those letters have an impact.

What will begin to happen is that you'll start paying more attention to your pangs. Soon you'll find yourself thinking about what letter you'll have to put after that food if you decide to eat it. You'll automatically run down the list of questions before you take that first bite. And the more practiced you become with being honest with yourself, the more often you'll reconsider eating something you shouldn't.

By the way, to help you remember which six questions to always ask yourself, just remember that the six letters (STIBAH) spell HABITS backward.

So why I didn't I just arrange the questions to spell the word out perfectly? Because I never want you to ask yourself if you're hungry first. If you did that, even if you weren't hungry, odds are you'd still say yes. But if you write down a different letter as you work through the first five questions, then most likely you were never hungry in the first place. Trust me!

The Eight That Elevate

Here's the deal: being smarter with my diet was a learning process for me. As a kid and throughout my entire basketball career I thought eating healthy meant having pretzels with no salt on them. But when you're young and constantly burning calories from participating in a sport as I was, you didn't have to be as considerate about the nutritional choices you're making.

But all that changed once I stopped playing professionally and got older. Being older and retired from pro sports naturally slowed my metabolism down, so I could no longer get away with what I was eating back then. Today I'm leaner in my forties than I was in my twenties, and it's not because I'm more active; it's because I realized how the mind, body, and spirit all work with one another and how eating to please all three was the key.

Nutrition isn't an easy landscape to navigate. We're tricked often into believing things are healthier for us than they really are. Thanks to all the fancy labels and clever packaging out there, it's hard to always know what's right for your body and know what's absolutely wrong to throw into it. But don't blame yourself: it turns out you're not alone. According to a study out of McGill University, the Nutrition Facts label currently on most food products in the United States and Canada is considered the least usable and most ineffective at improving smarter nutritional choices.[2]

That said, I do have a few principles that I apply to help you make that process a whole lot easier. If you follow these principles—these eight simple guidelines—you'll not only find yourself losing weight, building lean muscle, and feeling more energized, but your mind, body, and spirit will all rise as a result.

1. No Processed Foods

Once you embrace how meditation, exercise, and lifting your spirit make you feel better, boost your energy, and make you happier, you'll start to appreciate yourself more and start asking questions like, Do I really want to put something in my body that's capable of sitting on a shelf for a year?

Simply put, processed foods are any foods altered in some way to change their texture, make them last longer, or enhance their flavor. But what sounds more convenient and tasty usually equals added sugar or high-fructose corn syrup, trans and saturated fats, sodium, and monosodium glutamate (MSG). All those extra ingredients are typically behind weight gain, heart disease, and diabetes, but that's not stopping most people from eating them.

According to a recent study published in the *American Journal of Clinical Nutrition*, more than 75 percent of the foods purchased in US households is moderately processed (15.9 percent) or highly processed (61 percent).[3] When researchers broke those numbers down even further regarding convenience, ready-to-eat products (68.1 percent) and ready-to-heat (15.2 percent) products made up the bulk of purchases.

That's why this principle is at the top of my list. By eliminating them from your diet, you'll most likely be automatically removing three-quarters of the crap that's been holding you down.

But if you think this step is impossible, I understand. A lot of processed foods used to taste better to me too, until the first time I decided to step away from them for a little while. When I went back and tried them again—and I encourage you to do the same thing after your four weeks of LIFTED are up—I could taste the bad stuff in them and could literally feel them hurting my body. To this day the more real, fresh foods I eat, the more I immediately notice the negative effects that processed foods make on me when I eat them on rare occasions—and you will too.

2. Ingredients Count—Not Calories

I'll admit it—I used to calorie count. There was actually a time in my life when I was neurotic about the numbers. I remember those days well because I also remember how hungry I was all the time and that I never seemed to have a reliable amount of energy. I can also look back and admit that I wasn't eating any of the right kinds of foods that my body needed because I was looking at the numbers—not at the nutrients.

It really doesn't take a scientist to understand that if you put a Twinkie alongside an avocado, even though the avocado has more calories (289 calories for a single fruit, compared to 135 calories for one cake), it's nutritionally superior. In fact, it wouldn't even be a close race. And that's just one of the most basic and clearest examples I can give why calorie counting doesn't lead to healthy weight loss—it just leads to your body wanting more.

Instead, I want you to focus only on the ingredients in everything you eat.

Don't worry—I'm not expecting you to understand what all those ingredients mean. But that's the point. Before you eat something, turn the label around and start reading the ingredients from top to bottom. Then ask yourself, What is this ingredient doing for me? Then try that with each and every ingredient on the list.

Why I love this simple approach is threefold. One, you'll begin to educate yourself more about what's really in your foods as you find ingredients you don't even recognize and have to look up. Two, it makes you pause before eating bad things when you recognize that most of the additives don't have any benefit at all or might be bad for you in the first place. Finally, you'll find yourself turning to foods with far fewer ingredients because going through the process takes a lot of time. And to be honest, the fewer ingredients a food has listed, the more likely it is to be good for you in the first place. If you can't even understand what it is, do you really want to eat it?

But if you still feel the need to count something, try counting bites instead. When researchers at Brigham Young University had subjects count the number of bites they took every day, then asked them to take 20 to 30 percent fewer bites, subjects lost an average of four pounds—without changing a thing to their diet.[4]

3. Eat More Plants Than Animals

I've always believed that when you eat a plant-heavy diet, you really can't lose. Research has shown that eating just five portions of vegetables and fruit per day decreases your risk of death from any cause, ranging from cardiovascular disease to cancer.[5]

I'm not saying go vegan, as I understand that's a hard choice for a lot of people—and that's not how I eat anyway. My only strategy is that when you're putting together your meals, the biggest part of your plate should be vegetables.

If you're looking for answers to how much to eat or hoping for a certain number of grams or ounces to weigh out at every sitting, I have nothing for you because I don't do any of that micromanaging stuff. What I do try to do every meal is really as simple as this: my meals average about three-fourths veggies, then I fill the remaining space on my plate with a lean source of protein and a single serving of healthy fats.

Following this tried-and-true rule, you're always going to fill yourself up on fibrous vegetables. And if you're eating nothing but clean, organic vegetables, the list of vitamins, minerals, and other nutrients you'll bring into your body will be a roundup that most people's bodies never get to experience.

All that extra fiber and nutrients have a profound effect on your health, which is why science journals are filled with the positive effects of eating fruits and vegetables. But if you think it means gorging yourself or spending a lot of money, you'll be happy to know you don't need to do either. Research has shown that your risk of all-cause mortality (fancy talk for dying) decreases by 10 to 12 percent for every 50 cents extra you spend a day on fruits and vegetables.[6] In fact, studies have shown that those who eat just three servings of vegetables a day live an average of thirty-two months longer than people that never eat veggies.[7]

4. Minimize Your Grains

I used to eat a lot of carbs before a game, but the truth of the matter is that unless you're going out and running a 26.2-mile marathon the next day, I've never seen the point for anyone needing to carb load. Even when it's necessary before a big event, most people tend to overdo it.

Personally, I think that we can survive without grains. I live a grain-free life for the most part, or at least what I eat at home—I don't prepare grains for meals for myself.

Sure, if I'm having a great dinner someplace and grains are a part of the meal, I don't deny myself. But when you think about food from a fuel perspective, then you should look at your vegetables as your main source of fuel from carbohydrates.

If you're going to reach for grains, just be smart about choosing the ones that have more to offer you—and when you choose to eat them. When in doubt, try to eat only them after your workout (when your body can utilize them faster) and stick with whole-grain foods, which are made from the entire grain kernel, as opposed to refined grains, which have their bran and germ removed from them. Not only do whole grains digest at a slower pace than refined grains, which will leave you feeling fuller longer, but they are also richer in fiber, B vitamins, iron, and other essential nutrients that are important for your mind and body.

Some top choices to choose from: foods made from barley, cornmeal, oats, rye, and wheat, or whole grains such as brown rice, buckwheat, bulgur, millet, quinoa, rolled oats, and wild rice.

5. Give a High Five to Fat

When I was in college fat was bad, and pretty much everyone back then believed that so long as they were eating nonfat foods, they were fine. I wasn't any different, and every month when I'd buy snacks for my room, my entire wall would be filled with my go-to, fat-free foods: bottles of Mistic Juice and Twizzlers. And like any other normal college kid, I was drinking my fair share of alcohol. And not surprisingly, every month I'd wonder why my face was so chubby even though I wasn't eating anything fatty.

Today we're a little smarter about fat—or at least we should be. Yes, a gram of fat contains more than twice the amount of calories than a gram of protein and carbohydrates combined. But what you get back from unsaturated sources—both monounsaturated fats (MUFA) and polyunsaturated fats (PUFA)—far outweighs the calories you shouldn't be counting in the first place.

- **The bad fats that lower you:** Saturated fats (typically found in vegetable fats that remain liquid at room temperature, including palm and coconut oil, as well as meat, poultry skin, high-fat dairy, and eggs) and trans fats (found in fast foods, animal products, and anything that uses hydrogenated oil).

- **The good fats that LIFT you:** Nuts and seeds, all-natural nut butter, plant oils (such as flaxseed, canola, walnut, peanut, sunflower, sesame, soybean, and olive oil), cold-water fish, and avocados.

Getting the right amount of "good fats" in your diet not only stabilizes your blood sugar and lowers harmful LDL-cholesterol, but they also help lower your blood pressure, reduce inflammation, protect your organs, and provide fat-soluble vitamins, including A, D, E, and K.[8] But perhaps the best benefit of all is how you can immediately notice how healthy fats fill you up and satiate you right away. When I tell people to stay away from grains, they get nervous because they think they will never feel full throughout the day. The reality is that by having enough healthy fats in your diet, not only will you be less likely to feel hungry, but you'll find that you're more energized throughout the day as well.

So what's enough? Like I said, I'm not a calorie counter, even though the Institute of Medicine recommends that the average adult should consume 20 to 35 percent of their daily calories as fat. But a better way to gauge if you're getting enough is to shoot for four servings of healthy fats a day. Just a few examples of how much that would mean for you might include

- ½ ounce of any nuts or seeds
- 1 tablespoon of all-natural nut butter
- 1 tablespoon of a plant-based oil
- ¼ of an avocado
- 3 ounces of fatty fish (mackerel, salmon, or tuna, for example)

Do be careful with which healthy fats you choose. Nuts, for some people, can be a very tricky choice because of the amount of calories you can quickly consume if you're not careful. I've actually gained weight from those "secret healthy foods" that have found their way into my house in the past. There have been times when I've had nothing bad in my house but found myself eating two thousand calories worth of good food in a sitting just because it was so snackable. That's why when it comes to nuts, I prefer keeping those pack-size versions around instead of anything bought in bulk.

6. Eat Only Those Animals That Are Treated the Right Way

I eat meat, so I would never tell you not to. But if you're going to focus on eating healthy meats, I believe it's important also to focus on what the animals you eat are eating themselves. That's why no animal is off-limits in my program—chicken, fish, beef, pork—so long as it's hormone-free and free range.

You see, all my relatives come from farms in Kansas, so I grew up around farm animals and have a good understanding of what goes on at a good farm. My grandfather was a dairy farmer who truly cared about all of his cows and treated them well, so I could never imagine eating an animal that was treated inhumanely. Today my grandfather is in his late eighties and is still doing great, which I think speaks to the power of choosing to eat only those animals that have the best life possible.

One reason I feel strongly about eating this way is that it affects not just the animals' health but yours too. Studies have shown that animals that are inhumanely treated secrete more stress hormones. For example, hens under more distress tend to secrete more of the stress hormone corticosterone into the eggs they lay.[9] All those stress-induced hormones (which also includes adrenaline) not only change the taste of the meat by affecting its acidity but are transmitted to you when you eat animals that haven't been treated humanely.

But even if you don't subscribe to that theory, just look at it logically. Cows and pigs were never meant to be pumped full of hormones. They were also never meant to eat a grain-heavy diet because that's not the way their bodies evolved—they're supposed to be eating plants. So by breaking the food chain, doesn't it make you wonder what effect that has on you—the animal at the end of the food chain? If the meat you're eating is from animals that consumed foods they shouldn't, does it make any sense for you to be consuming them?

If you're still not on board, think of making the change as a spirit-boosting decision. I believe that if you're lifting yourself up by treating yourself and others with respect, it's important to have a broad approach to life and ask yourself, What effect am I having on the planet and everything that lives on it? Eating meats and fish that you know had the best life possible allows you to do just that.

7. Have Sweets in Moderation

If there's anything that I believe in, it's the importance of having a program that enhances the entire rest of your life. I would never deny your right to enjoy key lime pie if that's your favorite dessert in the whole world.

In fact, the whole LIFTED program is not a matter of giving up life's little pleasures—it's about eating the right types of foods that create a healthier body, which creates a healthier life, which ultimately creates happiness. It's about getting yourself to a place where you understand that when you eat something, you're making a decision at that moment—a decision that factors into a much larger formula that affects your mind, body, and spirit. And when you start seeing these little decisions as rewarding or seeing them as small victories, then you'll notice that you'll find happiness in them instead of looking at them as a hater.

That said, I'll admit it—I love key lime pie, and I enjoy ice cream three times a week. But when I eat it, I eat it in moderation and choose a brand that's made from the least amount of ingredients possible (five or fewer) versus some synthetic form of dessert pumped with artificial sweeteners just because it's lower in calories.

The entire reason most people use artificial sweeteners is to save calories, but does it make sense to eat something unnatural to save a few calories? Instead, I believe that the more you can get a sweetener in its natural state, the less of a negative impact it will make on your body. Most artificial sweeteners have been shown to trigger the release of insulin, increase your appetite, raise your risk of developing type II diabetes, and boost your need for sweeter and sweeter foods.[10]

So my challenge for the next four weeks is this: step away from all artificial sweeteners. Instead, when you find it necessary to sweeten food, use things that are all-natural and as close to the earth as possible. After you've gone through the four-week program, let yourself have a serving and see how your stomach feels—and watch it blow up! I guarantee you that after a month, you will actually witness the way your body rejects them. Once you start having that experience of actually noticing the way artificial sweeteners affect your body, it will shift your perspective about using them as regularly as you might right now.

- **The bad sweets that lower you:** Anything made with saccharin, sucralose, aspartame, neotame, acesulfame potassium, and erythritol.
- **The good sweets that LIFT you:** Unfiltered honey, coconut sugar, date sugar, stevia, and maple syrup.

8. Eat Clean, But Don't Be Cleaned Out

Following the Eight That Elevate tips will have you automatically eating a clean diet, but my final tip is less of a what-to-eat as much as it's a what-not-to-waste-your-time-eating tip.

Ideally, eating only organic foods will lower your risk of ingesting toxins, pesticides, chemicals, and other contaminants that are more widespread than ever in many foods out there. But I also get annoyed in grocery stores when I see things like "organic bananas," "organic cantaloupes," or other fruits and vegetables that don't need to be organic because they either have a thicker protective skin or aren't as attractive to insects or other harmful things so they aren't treated with chemicals as often. If you're looking to save a buck, check out ewg.org for their "clean fifteen" and "dirty dozen" lists (they are updated annually). The following don't necessarily need to be organic to be okay by me:

asparagus	kiwi
avocados	mangoes
broccoli	onions
cabbage	papayas
cantaloupe	pineapples
eggplant	sweet peas
grapefruit	sweet corn
honeydew	

Beyond the Eight:
What Works for Me—And Might Work for You

I've always found it interesting how nutrition advice has changed over the years. I watched experts recommend everything from breaking down each meal into 30 percent protein, 30 percent fat, and 40 percent carb portions to suggesting the trick is to fast for thirteen hours. I've been told to eat like a Mediterranean, dine like a cavewoman, shy away from carbs completely, and avoid foods cooked or heated above 118 degrees Fahrenheit.

So which is the right way to eat—and which is the wrong way?

As I said at the start of this chapter, this isn't a diet book, and I don't think everything works for everybody—but I know what works for me. That said, here are just a few other ways I stay LIFTED nutritionally all day long. Look at them as sort of a loose working outline of things I believe in, and if you can dial into a few that work for you, then be prepared to soar even higher toward your goals.

Make Sure Every Meal Pleases All Three

Sometimes, deciding what to eat when LIFTING yourself can be as easy as asking

- What will this meal do for my mind?
- What will this meal do for my body?
- What will this meal do for my spirit?

If all three answers are nothing but positive, odds are you're probably eating because you're actually hungry and making smart, nutritional choices. But if you can't answer any of the questions or you answer any or all in a negative way, you may want to rethink what you're about to snack on. In other words, if all three answers are positive, you'll be LIFTING all three. If not, you're most likely holding yourself down.

What's Good for All *May Not Be Good for* You

Over the last two years something that's been a big game-changer for me has been trusting my body a bit more. You've seen them—those lists of healthy foods that are wonderful because they have the right nutritional mix. But the thing is, don't believe every "good-for-you" food is always the best choice for *your* body.

Take eggs, for example. Nothing offers more nutritional value in terms of protein than an egg, and when I was in my twenties, I used to eat two hard-boiled eggs fifteen minutes before I exercised. But for some reason I'm not able to digest whole eggs like I used to. If I have them, I suddenly feel full and lousy for hours. But when I was first starting to experience that reaction, I never equated it to eating eggs and blamed it on other foods. After all—eggs were on the "good" list.

Here's the thing: we all process food differently. One landmark study performed by the Weizmann Institute of Science in Israel tracked the blood-sugar levels of eight hundred people to see how their bodies responded to eating the same foods over a week's time.[11] A total of roughly forty-seven thousand meals were measured—and guess what? The data showed that different people had vastly different responses to the same food, so we don't all metabolize food—even if it's incredibly healthy for us—in the same way.

That's why it's important to pay attention to how your body reacts to every type of food. When you dial into your body like this, you do yourself a service because you won't just be blindly following the rules on what you should and shouldn't eat. Something might be healthy, but if the way your body reacts to it isn't healthy, then take it off the list—even if it's one of the healthiest things you can eat—then find an alternative food that offers similar benefits regarding its nutrients.

Don't Settle for Snack Food

I feel blessed to live in New York for many reasons, and one of them is that I can get whatever type of snack I want right around every corner. But if you're in the car and on the go or you need to have something in your office or your bag at all times, I understand there are limitations. The main thing to remember is that when you need an afternoon snack, it doesn't have to be a snack food.

In other words, why settle for snack food when it's snack time?

That's where a lot of people get themselves in trouble. They'll eat healthy when it's mealtime, but snacks somehow become a free-for-all. Even hearing the word *snack* may sometimes be the reason you're reaching for things that are less nutritious in the first place. Maybe it's because we've been led to believe that anything we eat in between meals needs to be some sort of grab-and-go option or something with less flair like an apple with a little peanut butter on it, when that's not the case at all.

You don't have to back yourself into a snack corner; instead, you can continue to eat the same types of meals you're having for breakfast, lunch, or dinner—only make them smaller. A lot of times I'll just wrap up what's left of my lunch and have that final quarter around three o'clock. Or I might have a small container of beets and diced chicken. My point being, if you find yourself reaching for the wrong foods in between meals, try making a little extra of the good foods you're having during mealtime so you have a few convenient smaller-sized portions around to eat instead.

Water First—Wants Second

Often after a spin class I'll be craving a coconut water or find myself wanting to reach for watermelon juice. But if I drink water first, then I'll usually notice that my desire for what I originally wanted to drink goes away. I'll actually say to myself, "You know what? I'm good now!" That's why I always put water front and center before any other craving I might have when I want something to drink.

Need another reason or two? When researchers at the University of Illinois at Urbana-Champaign examined the nutritional habits of more than eighteen thousand adults, they found that the majority of subjects who increased their consumption of water by just 1 percent—1 percent!—reduced their total daily calorie intake along with their daily intake of sugar, sodium, saturated fat, and cholesterol.[12] In addition, those who drank an extra one to three cups of water daily ate between 68 to 205 fewer calories and 78 to 235 mg less sodium a day.

I get that water can be boring, although there are ways to make it better, like putting fruit in your water (such as cucumbers or berries) and letting it sit to change the taste a little bit. But reaching for juice or anything with calories and/or sugar when you're really thirsty can be a big pitfall for many people. Instead, try having at least one full glass of water first to see if that sends the craving away.

If it doesn't, that's fine, so long as you remain mindful of how much sugar is in whatever drink you're reaching for. If I'm not in the mood for water and just not having it, then I'm a big fan of maple water. For me, it's just enough to satisfy, but it's low in sugar.

I also love smoothies, but you need to be able to navigate the menu or else it's easy to drink more calories than your body really needs. I have a Vitamix at home and often make my own smoothies. My rules—for smoothies I buy or make—are simple:

- Only use one fruit, because adding any more than that can turn that drink into a sugar bomb!
- Stick with low-glycemic fruits, such as strawberries, blueberries, or pears.
- Whatever amount of fruit you *think* you need, try using half as much. You really don't need a lot of fruit to taste their flavor. So sometimes, instead of one banana, I'll use half or ask for just half if I'm buying a smoothie.
- Add protein if possible. I recommend adding dairy-free varieties, such as vegan or collagen protein.
- Finally, throw in some greens—spinach and kale are my favorites. If that sounds disgusting, definitely don't knock it until you've tried it. Use a milder green like spinach or Romaine, and seriously, you will not even taste it. Trust me: I challenge you to mix a handful of greens with a half-banana, some almond milk, and a scoop of protein—the taste just might surprise you.

Look for the Little Cheerleaders
Along the Way

Maybe your main reason to try LIFTED was to finally be a little lighter on the scale. But by simply following the Eight That Elevate, you'll automatically be eating a cleaner, healthier diet that will change other things about you from head to toe simultaneously.

Along the way don't be surprised when you start noticing that you're sleeping more soundly, have a nicer smile, feel more alert, or notice your mood improving. A recent study published in the *British Journal of Health Psychology* found that just by eating fruits and vegetables, you will feel happier, more creative, and more curious.[13]

One thing you may notice right away is a change in your skin, particularly when it comes to bloating. When you eat poorly for a long time, you get used to being bloated, and I think there's nothing worse in the world than feeling bloated. But when I eat right my skin becomes naturally tighter, and if you don't know that you're missing out on that, you don't know how good that feels not to be that way.

It's these perks along the path that sometimes go unnoticed, but they are your little cheerleaders. These are the things you may not necessarily think about, but when you recognize them, you realize there are these little bonuses along the way. When you can dial into these little things, they cheer you along and keep you going when the big picture gets a little daunting. So take time to notice when you have more energy, or when your skin looks amazing one day, or that you don't feel bloated. Stay mindful, realize that no little thing like that is too small, and look at each as a victorious moment along your journey.

For the Last Three, Use the Three Ts

In basketball it's often the last few minutes of the game when the game is either won or lost. That same truism applies to your diet. When it comes to healthy eating, a lot of people can maintain their diet from morning until just around those last three hours before they head to bed. But once they reach that three-hour zone, that's when everything falls apart.

It's that uncontrollable evening eating that most people have a hard time with—and I'm no different. Because I'm busy and look at my food as fuel during the day, it's somewhat easier to eat clean. But something happens in those magical last few hours of the night when I'm the most tired and least distracted. That's when it's so easy to take an entirely good day and throw it all away—when twelve hours of willpower gets destroyed by three hours of weakness.

How do I keep myself in check for those last three hours of the night when most people tend to fail? I've always relied on three tactics to make it through unscathed:

- **Teeth:** Something I've done over the years that works for me is instead of brushing my teeth at bedtime, I brush them once I'm done eating for the night. Using this trick usually keeps me from wanting to eat again because, on those rare occasions when I have, it makes me feel lousy knowing I'll have to brush them all over again.

- **Tea:** A lot of times the reason we snack at night is that we're winding down from the rest of our day and just looking for something to do. So all your late-night eating may be just the act of needing to do something. That's why I found just the whole ritual of making and drinking tea (something caffeine-free—I prefer chamomile) to be a great way to satiate that need without eating anything my body shouldn't be having unnecessarily as a result.

- **Talk:** Believe it or not, whether I'm by myself or other people are over, I'll actually say out loud that "the kitchen is closed!" Yep, I'll make an official proclamation that the room containing all my food is now off-limits. I'll admit that sometimes this doesn't work as well as the other two do, but when you make yourself accountable—even if it's just to yourself—it can leave you feeling like you're going back on your word, which I've found makes me less likely to do it.

If You're Bored, You Haven't Explored

When I tell clients what I eat and how at least three-quarters of my plate are leafy greens and vegetables (with the rest of my plate filled with lean protein), I've had some say that's boring. But if you look at the infinite number of ways you can have vegetables and you're still bored, well, then . . . you're probably just not doing it right.

I encourage all my clients to venture out and explore the thousands of different vegetables out there so they can open their world up to all possibilities—and not just the few dozen vegetables they typically stick with. But just in case you're not ready to be adventurous with the unknown, I called on the culinary expertise of Carolyn Brown, MS, RD, a nutritionist at Foodtrainers, a private practice in New York, where she specializes in individualized weight-management plans. In no time her creativity and nutritional know-how dreamt up a few veggie-heavy recipes that are as easy to assemble as they are incredibly delicious. Because of Carolyn, there's no excuse not to LIFT your meals to the next level, so thank her by following her on Instagram (@carolynbrownnutrition) after you try a few of these recipes on for size!

Should You Eat Before You Exercise?

Maybe—it depends on you. When I was in college, my coaches would plan our pregame meal exactly three hours before the game. That meal would be free of a lot of spices and had the perfect amount of carbohydrates and protein so we had sustained energy from the time the game began until long after the game was over. I was lucky enough to have someone looking out for me, someone who understood that what I ate *before* I was active had a major effect on what I could do—or how I felt—*while* I was active.

Today, when I teach my morning spin classes, I'm performing 500 to 700 calorie pushes. They're intense, so when I eat the wrong things or I don't eat enough, I can physically feel when my tank is empty. But what works best for me is having my coffee and eating something small (like a pack of blackberries) just to put something in my stomach. After that, I have all the energy I need from that small serving and whatever I ate from the night before to make it through teaching two hours of spin.

But that's me.

The best solution falls somewhere in the middle. Is there any truth that exercising while in a fasted state will cause your body to utilize more fat as energy so you burn more body fat? Absolutely! But for some of you not having anything in the tank before exercising could prevent you from working out as long or as intensely, leaving you less likely to see as many results for all of your efforts.

A good rule of thumb, if you feel you have the energy to go through your workout, then great. But ask yourself afterward, Did I perform well? Was I able to give it all that I could give? If not, you may be the type that needs to eat a little something before a workout, so have something at least forty-five minutes to an hour before you work out so that your digestive process has already begun. That way your body won't be putting energy toward digestion that could be going toward your workout.

My recommendation: a nice mix of protein and carbohydrates, like a half-banana and a tablespoon of peanut butter, or an egg white with a piece of fruit. The more you get LIFTED, the more you'll be able to read your body's cues. It's talking to you all the time.

Should You Eat After You Exercise?

Yes! If you're the type who thinks it's counterproductive to eat after exercise because the entire reason you're working out in the first place is to lose weight, then stop being that type right now.

I understand the struggle in rethinking the way you've been programmed to think, because I used to be that girl too. But if you think of your body as a machine and food as fuel, then you need to understand physiologically what's going on after you exercise. Whether you want to visualize it or not, what strength training does is break down and tear apart muscle tissue—muscle tissue that needs to be rebuilt if you want to keep and build more lean muscle that will ignite your metabolism so you're burning fat all day long.

Eating within an hour after your workout is crucial to making that happen, but you need to have the right mix of nutrients being put to work. The best ratio for your body is a three-to-one carbs-to-protein mix, so aim for about 30 to 45 grams of carbs and 10 to 15 grams of protein (which amounts to roughly only 160 to 220 calories). Give or take, that's the right amount to give your muscles the amino acids to rebuild muscle along with enough carbohydrates to refill your glycogen (the stored carbohydrates in your muscles and liver that your body uses along with stored body fat when you exercise).

To be honest, I'm not a big fan of protein shakes, but it depends on your lifestyle. If that's the only way you can get something into your body right away, then do it. However, I would recommend a nondairy form of protein, such as pea, soy, brown rice, or collagen—and one that has the cleanest ingredients.

Otherwise, one of your biggest meals of the day should come after your workout. It's really a magic hour when your metabolism's still elevated and your body makes the most out of everything you eat. To take advantage of that time, make sure you're getting a decent amount of protein (three to four ounces of a lean protein source), at least three-fourths of a plate of vegetables or leafy greens, along with a serving of fruit or some honey, which provides enough of a simple sugar source that your body can convert it into glycogen.

THE RECIPES

Breakfast

Awesome Avo-Baked-Eggs

SERVES 2

1 large ripe avocado
2 organic eggs (pasture raised are ideal)
¼ teaspoon pepper

2 tablespoons chopped chives
pinch of salt to taste
½ cup side of fruit, optional

1. Preheat the oven to 425°F.
2. Slice the avocado in half, and remove the pit. Scoop out about two tablespoons of flesh from the center of each half of the avocado, just enough so the egg will fit right in the center. (You can save the avocado flesh to spread on a wrap or add to a smoothie.)
3. Place the avocado in a small baking dish. Do your best to make sure the halves fit tightly so they don't tilt over.
4. Crack an egg into each half of the avocado. Try to put the yolk in first, then let the egg whites spill in to fill up the rest of the avocado space.
5. Place in the oven, and bake for 15 to 20 minutes. Cooking time depends on the size of the egg and avocado, but be sure the egg whites have enough time to cook through.
6. Remove your avo-egg from the oven, then season with pepper and chives. Serve with fruit on the side if desired.

Calories per serving: 190; Protein: 7 grams; Fat: 16 grams; Carbs: 7 grams

Zesty Coconut Parfait

SERVES 1

½ cup coconut yogurt
½ teaspoon vanilla extract
a few drops of stevia, optional
1 cup blueberries

1 tablespoon hemp seeds
1 tablespoon chopped almonds
1 tablespoon coconut flakes
1 teaspoon lemon zest

1. Stir yogurt, vanilla extract, and stevia (if using) together.
2. Top with blueberries, hemp seeds, almonds, and coconut flakes. (If you feel like getting fancy, alternate these in layers with the yogurt in a clear serving dish.)
3. Sprinkle on the lemon zest, and dig in!

Calories per serving: 270; Protein: 4 grams; Fat: 21 grams; Carbs: 18 grams

Fantastic Herb Frittata

SERVES 4 TO 5

6 organic eggs, beaten (pasture raised are ideal)
¾ teaspoon turmeric
½ teaspoon Himalayan or other sea salt
1 cup chopped scallions
1 garlic clove, chopped

3 cups of any combo of chopped herbs (use what you have—1 cup each of dill, parsley, and cilantro work well; basil is also a winner)
2 tablespoons ghee or coconut oil

1. Preheat the oven to 400°F.
2. Whisk eggs together with turmeric and salt. Add scallions, garlic, and herbs, and stir to combine.
3. Heat the oil in an oven-safe pan (I like cast iron) over medium flame.
4. Add egg/herb mixture and cook for 3 to 4 minutes, until beginning to harden.
5. Transfer pan to oven, and cook 7 to 10 minutes or until firm and not runny.
6. Slice into 4 to 5 pieces. You can refrigerate or freeze leftovers. It works cold the next day with greens and makes a great travel meal too.

Calories per serving: 350; Protein: 13 grams; Fat: 20 grams; Carbs: 19 grams

Zap Your Appetite Smoothie

SERVES 1

1 cup unsweetened coconut milk
½ cup blueberries (frozen are fine)
½ banana
1 tablespoon plant-based protein powder
1 tablespoon coconut oil or ½ avocado

5 drops stevia
¼ teaspoon peppermint extract
ice
handful of spinach, optional
handful of fresh mint, optional

1. Add all ingredients to blender, and blend until smooth.

2. Pour into a glass and enjoy!

Calories per serving: 390; Protein: 22 grams; Fat: 18 grams; Carbs: 48 grams

Excellent Avocado Sweet Potato "Toast"

SERVES 2

1 sweet potato
1 avocado
2 teaspoons extra-virgin olive oil

pinch Himalayan sea salt
red pepper flakes

1. Slice sweet potato into four ¼-thick slices, and pop into the toaster until cooked through. This may take a few rounds of toasting and as long as 15 minutes, depending on your toaster power. (You can also use your oven. Just set it to 400°F and bake for 30 minutes—15 minutes for each side).

2. Open and pit the avocado, and then slice into slivers or mash up into avocado mash.

3. Top the sweet potato with avocado. Drizzle with oil, then top with salt and red pepper flakes.

Calories per serving: 210; Protein: 2 grams; Fat: 16 grams; Carbs: 18 grams

Lunch

ABC De-licious Salad (Avocado-Basil-Chicken)

SERVES 3

2 boneless, skinless, organic chicken breasts, cooked, or 1/2 organic rotisserie chicken, shredded or cubed

½ cup fresh basil leaves, stems removed

1 large ripe avocado, pit and skin removed

1 tablespoon extra-virgin olive oil

¼ teaspoon turmeric

½ teaspoon sea salt, or more to taste

⅛ teaspoon ground black pepper, or more to taste

1. Place the chicken in a medium mixing bowl.
2. Combine the basil, avocado, oil, turmeric, salt, and pepper in a food processor or blender, and blend until smooth. You may need to scrape the sides down to ensure it's all mixed in.
3. Pour the basil mix into the mixing bowl with the chicken, and toss well to coat.
4. Taste, and add any additional salt and ground pepper if needed.
5. Refrigerate until ready to serve. Note: the avocado dressing may turn brown by the next day (you can add a squeeze of lemon to help this slightly), but it's still good to eat!

Calories per serving: 200; Protein: 18 grams; Fat: 13 grams; Carbs: 4 grams

Miso Happy Salad

SERVES 1

Miso Dressing

½ tablespoon miso
1 tablespoon apple cider vinegar
2 tablespoons extra-virgin olive oil
dash turmeric
dash black pepper

Salad

2 cups dark greens, such as Tuscan kale, chard, spinach, arugula, or any green mix
½ avocado
1 tablespoon pumpkin seeds (AKA pepitas)
4 ounces wild salmon, grilled
optional toppings: sliced asparagus, radishes, fennel, carrots, bell peppers, cucumbers

1. Add all dressing ingredients in a small jar with a lid; cover and shake until all are well combined.
2. Combine all salad ingredients in a bowl, and top with the dressing. Enjoy!

Calories per serving: 700; Protein: 35 grams; Fat: 57 grams; Carbs: 15 grams

Simple Lemon-Basil Shrimp

SERVES 2

1 lemon
¾ to 1 pound large raw shrimp, cleaned
1 tablespoon extra-virgin olive oil, coconut oil, or ghee
1 garlic clove, minced
salt and pepper to taste

2 cups fresh basil, cut into strips (cilantro also works well here. Either way, reserve some whole, pretty leaves for garnish.)
red pepper flakes or hot sauce
greens, microgreens, or zucchini noodles (page 178), to serve

1. Use a vegetable peeler on the lemon to zest 6 strips off of it. Cut the remaining lemon in half.

(Continues)

(*Continued*)

Simple Lemon-Basil Shrimp

2. Place the shrimp on a plate with a paper towel, and make sure they are dry (they will sear better dry than wet).
3. Heat a pan to medium-high, and add oil to the pan. Once hot, add the shrimp, followed by the lemon zest, garlic, and salt and pepper, and cook for 4 minutes.
4. Once the shrimp are thoroughly cooked, squeeze the juice from the remaining half-lemon into the pan, and turn off the heat.
5. Add the basil and red pepper flakes, and serve over zucchini noodles or greens.

Calories per serving: 240; Protein: 32 grams; Fat: 10 grams; Carbs: 5 grams

Zucchini Noodles with Paleo Pesto

SERVES 2

2 zucchinis
1 tablespoon extra-virgin olive oil
Paleo Pesto (see next page)

4 ounces organic grilled chicken or fish, optional

1. Peel the zucchinis into ribbons or zucchini spaghetti using a spiralizer, mandolin, or vegetable peeler.
2. Heat oil in a medium pan over medium heat. Add the zucchini ribbons, and cook for 2 to 3 minutes.
3. Top with Paleo Pesto and chicken or fish, if using.

Paleo Pesto

SERVES 2

⅓ cup pine nuts or raw sunflower seeds
1 garlic clove, smashed with the side of a knife
2 cups fresh basil

½ cup extra-virgin olive oil
1½ tablespoons lemon juice
½ teaspoon sea salt
¼ teaspoon black pepper

1. Pulse the pine nuts and garlic in a food processor or blender until evenly chopped. Add the basil, and continue to pulse.
2. With the blender running, add the oil, juice, salt, and pepper, and blend until smooth.
3. Use the pesto immediately over Zucchini Noodles, or refrigerate for up to 4 to 5 days.

Calories per serving: 410; Protein: 4 grams; Fat: 42 grams; Carbs: 9 grams

Chicken Lettuce "Mock-o Tacos"

SERVES 4

1 head butter lettuce
2 tablespoons extra-virgin olive oil
1 pound boneless, skinless chicken breasts, cut into small pieces
3 tablespoons organic taco seasoning

optional toppings: 1 tomato, diced small; ½ cup red bell pepper, diced small; ¼ cup fresh cilantro leaves, finely chopped; ½ cup canned (BPA-free) black beans, drained and rinsed; 1 avocado, peeled and diced; your favorite salsa

1. Peel leaves off the head of butter lettuce, and set aside—these will be your taco shells.
2. Heat a large pan to medium-high heat, and add the oil and chicken, cooking about 4 minutes. Sprinkle in seasoning, and stir to coat evenly for 2 minutes until

(Continues)

(*Continued*)

Chicken Lettuce "Mock-o Tacos"

the chicken is well coated and thoroughly cooked through, just beginning to brown. Remove from heat.

3. Place a lettuce leaf on a plate, and build your "taco," adding about 3 tablespoons chicken, followed by your choice of toppings.

4. Fold up and eat, and repeat! If you're finding that the lettuce wraps fall apart easily, use two at a time.

Calories per serving (with toppings added): 580; Protein: 60 grams; Fat: 28 grams; Carbs: 26 grams

Dinner

Spicy Secret Weapon Salmon

SERVES 4

1 pound wild salmon, skin and bones
    removed, cut into 4 pieces
1 tablespoon coconut oil
½ teaspoon turmeric
¼ teaspoon cayenne or hot sauce

juice from ½ lemon
Himalayan sea salt
2 cups veggies (some great options to
    try: Brussels sprouts, asparagus, or
    greens), optional

1. Preheat the oven to 425°F.
2. Combine oil, turmeric, cayenne, juice, and salt in a small bowl.
3. Place salmon on a baking sheet lined with parchment paper. Brush or spread the oil mixture on top of the salmon.
4. Bake for 15 minutes. (If the salmon is thick, it may need a little extra time.)
5. Serve with veggies, if using.

Calories per serving: 190; Protein: 23 grams; Fat: 11 grams; Carbs: less than 1 gram

Simply Succulent Zucchini Soup

SERVES 4

3 tablespoons extra-virgin olive oil
1 small onion, finely chopped
2 garlic cloves, thinly sliced
Himalayan sea salt
freshly ground black pepper
2 pounds zucchini, chopped into
¼-inch-thick pieces

1 cup vegetable stock or low-sodium,
organic chicken broth
optional toppings: zucchini slivers;
pumpkin seeds; avocado,
thinly sliced

1. Heat the oil in a large saucepan over low-medium heat. Add the onion and garlic, seasoning lightly with salt and pepper. Stir frequently for 6 to 7 minutes, until the garlic and onion are soft.
2. Add the zucchini, and cook until softened, about 10 minutes.
3. Add the stock and 1½ cups of water, bring to a simmer, and cook until zucchini is completely soft.
4. Carefully pour the soup into blender, and puree it in batches until it's a silky-smooth consistency and bright green in color. Season with salt and pepper to taste, and serve either hot or cold, garnished with zucchini slivers, pumpkin seeds, or avocado slices.

Calories per serving: 140; Protein: 3 grams; Fat: 11 grams; Carbs: 11 grams

Spicy Thai Carrot Noodles

SERVES 1

Noodles
1 large carrot,
 washed and peeled

Sunflower Thai dressing

1 tablespoon sunbutter
2 teaspoons extra-virgin olive oil
2 teaspoons lemon juice
1 teaspoon raw apple cider vinegar
¼ teaspoon minced fresh ginger
salt and pepper to taste
red pepper flakes or scallion for garnish,
 optional

1. Use spiralizer or julienne peeler to make "noodles" with the carrot.
2. Combine all dressing ingredients in a blender or with a small whisk. If it's super-thick, add a splash of water or an extra few drops of oil.
3. Toss carrot noodles with sunbutter mixture. Eat right away, or refrigerate until ready to eat.

Calories per serving: 220; Protein: 3 grams; Fat: 20 grams; Carbs: 11 grams

Savory Pesto Turkey Sliders Over Greens

SERVES 4

1 pound organic ground turkey
 (or chicken or salmon)
2 tablespoons Paleo Pesto (page 179)
1 garlic clove, minced

pinch salt
freshly ground black pepper
greens, for serving

1. Combine all the ingredients in a large bowl. Form into 4 patties.
2. Grill for 10 to 12 minutes, flipping once. Serve over greens.

Calories per serving: 330; Protein: 26 grams; Fat: 25 grams; Carbs: less than 1 gram

Pistachi-Oh-Yes! Crusted Chicken

You will never miss breaded chicken with this pistachio-crusted deliciousness.

SERVES 4

3 ounces coconut yogurt

1 cup loosely packed cilantro, plus more for garnish

2 tablespoons lemon juice, plus wedges for serving

½ tablespoon ground cumin

½ tablespoon salt

4 thin chicken cutlets

¾ cup shelled pistachios (unsalted is ideal, but okay if not), finely ground in food processor

2 teaspoons extra-virgin olive oil w

8 spears steamed asparagus, for serving

1. Heat oven to 350ºF.
2. Puree in a food processer the yogurt, cilantro, garlic, juice, cumin, and salt until smooth (and bright green!). Transfer the yogurt mixture to a large resealable bag. Add the chicken, seal the bag, and shake well until coated.
3. Spread pistachios on a wide plate. Remove the chicken from the yogurt mixture, and drag through the pistachio crumbs, pressing until fully coated. Shake off any excess.
4. Heat oil over medium-high heat in a large, oven-proof skillet. Cook the chicken until golden brown, flipping after 1 to 2 minutes. Carefully transfer the pan to the preheated oven to finish cooking the chicken. Bake until it's cooked completely through, about 5 minutes.
5. Serve over the asparagus, and garnish with extra cilantro and lemon wedges.

Calories per serving: 460; Protein: 38 grams; Fat: 27 grams; Carbs: 14 grams

Snacks

Apple-Almond Butter Rings

SERVES 1

1 medium organic apple, cored and
    sliced into rings
2 tablespoons almond butter

1 tablespoon dark chocolate chips
sprinkle of cinnamon

1. Spread almond butter onto an apple slice, then sprinkle with chocolate chips and cinnamon. Top with remaining the apple slice, pressing down gently to make the sandwiches.

Calories per serving: 350; Protein: 7 grams; Fat: 22 grams; Carbs: 39 grams

Choco-Espresso Protein Smoothie

SERVES 1

½ cup unsweetened almond milk
½ banana
1 tablespoon almond butter
1 tablespoon cocoa powder
1 scoop chocolate plant-based protein
   powder

2 teaspoons instant espresso coffee
   (or any instant coffee)
1 teaspoon vanilla extract
1 cup ice
stevia, optional

1. Add all ingredients to a blender, and blend until smooth.
2. Pour into a glass, and enjoy!

Calories per serving: 270; Protein: 16 grams; Fat: 13 grams; Carbs: 29 grams

Turkey Rev-Up Roll-Ups

SERVES 1

4 to 5 organic turkey slices
2 to 3 large lettuce or kale leaves

½ avocado, cut into slices
mustard, optional

1. Place 1 to 2 turkey slices in each lettuce leaf, top with the avocado and mustard, if using. Roll up, and snack away!

Calories per serving (with mustard): 230; Protein: 15 grams; Fat: 12 grams; Carbs: 11 grams

7

How to LIFT Yourself Higher

Just because you've finished the four-week LIFTED program doesn't mean your journey is over. There's a saying I use in my classes:

This moment becomes a day. This day becomes a week. This week becomes a month. This month becomes a season. And this season becomes your life. *That* is how important this moment is.

You see, this was never about four weeks. This is a book about life. It's about how you can be your happiest and healthiest but still be able to live the life you want. This is about giving you the tools that will allow you to LIFT yourself for a lifetime. And if you don't think you can do it, then here's something I share with those who have taken the journey with me but doubt they can find that greatness within themselves again:

If you're not sure you can—then you MUST.
Do not start to negotiate with yourself—not now. You've come too far.
You were given this life because you are strong enough to live it.

It's time to keep living your life to its fullest—starting today. Now here's how we're going to do it together.

Seize the Celebration
for Two Straight Days

First things first: the day after you've completed the four-week LIFTED program—I'm serious . . . the very moment it's over—I want you to take a breath and give yourself the time to feel proud of yourself and savor what you've achieved.

Something we're all so quick to do—and I used to do the same thing after I would win a championship—is to cut our celebratory time short. Too quickly I would focus on how to prepare for the next season. But this moment—this was what the entire journey was all about, do you understand? As much as we want to set goals for ourselves and reach our dreams, life is all about balance. It's all about being thankful and proud of ourselves.

That's why I want you to take two days off as well as celebrate this victory by treating yourself to something.

The only thing I don't want is you to reward yourself with food or alcohol. These two days are about celebrating getting your life on track, so the last thing I need you to do is reach for the same foods or vices you've been trying to get away from or bring under control.

Instead, try to reward yourself with something that's different from your usual approach to celebration. Maybe that means a spa day or a weekend away somewhere. Maybe it's just something as small—but significant—as taking the afternoon off from work to go to the park and listen to some music. I want you to do something you might not necessarily do for yourself all the time.

Even if you choose not to reward yourself, you *need* that moment for yourself. Remember in the first place, this entire four-week journey was about *this moment*, so you're cheating yourself if you just skip over it and don't acknowledge. In between goals is this little thing called life—so enjoy every moment!

How to LIFT Yourself to the Next Level

Once you've rejoiced in completing the LIFTED program for two days, it's time to LIFT yourself all over again. I don't feel you need any more than two days off. After all, you should continue and stay in the zone because this zone is your new life.

You could repeat the same four-week program again to the letter if you like. And if you're new to exercise or just want to experience LIFTED in the exact same way as you did before—because it brought so much joy into your life—that's fine. So long as each time you feel LIFTED by the program and find yourself on track toward your goals, there's no pressure to change things at all.

But once you're ready to see how much further you can fly, all it takes is reassessing your goals and your Dream Board along with tweaking what to do during the mind, body, and spirit portions of the program. If that sounds like a lot of work, I promise you that it's not. All you need to do is set aside a few minutes for yourself. And if you do, if you take the time to spend a few moments asking yourself the right questions (which I'll show you in this chapter), the amazing feeling you just experienced by completing the program is about to become even more magnificent.

Speaking as a former pro athlete, whenever we started a new season or it was time to play against someone I had played against before, I took the time to reevaluate and rethink my plan of attack. That meant looking back on what I had done, reconsidering the choices I had made, and remembering which mistakes I had made. It was about where I was then versus where I am now. It's called strategy.

After all, it would be silly not to evaluate how well we did as a team or how poorly we played to figure out what to do for the next time. It made things easier to decide whether the best approach was to stick with the same plan and just put more effort into it—or change things up entirely.

The same principles apply to repeating the LIFTED program. If you don't continually evaluate yourself, you'll never get as much from it as you could. But to do that, you need to be completely honest with yourself about what's possible. That means looking at yourself through a realistic lens based on what you've done up until this point and what you noticed along the way.

Before You Start

In the next section I'll show you what to tweak with every part of the program. But right now I just want you to ask yourself the following three questions:

Did I Give It My All?

Ask yourself, Is *this* it? Is *this* what I'm giving myself today? Is what I put into the program for four weeks all that I could have put into it? And will I give myself more the next time through?

I want your answers to reflect that you tried your absolute best and that you'll try your absolute best the next time, and the next time, and the time after that. You need to be in the mindset of always wanting to try your best and always giving your all. Because if you're not in that zone, if you're not dialed into that attitude, you'll LIFT yourself only so far, no matter how many times you try the program.

Did Something Get in My Way?

If so, then that's okay. Life happens, and something I always say is, "My yesterday does not define my today." And if it was you that got in your own way, the same rule applies. I don't want you to ever interpret your mistakes as failures; instead, be willing to make mistakes. Fall down! Life isn't meant to be lived perfectly; it's about how well we dust ourselves off and stand up again.

Here's the thing: Mistakes are *proof* that you are trying, and that's all that matters. That's all that matters to me, and it should be all that matters to you.

Throughout my entire career I have had tons of failures—and I have had thousands of highs and lows. Yet one thing I always kept was focus. I always knew where I was going. But I get it: when I suffered certain failures after basketball, I felt mortal. I felt scared. But sometimes when things are falling apart, they may be falling into place. The important thing is that you finished it. And you know what? You'll do it again.

Did Something Give Me Momentum?

I believe that life gives us gifts, and one of those gifts is momentum. There is great power in momentum, and when you have momentum, you need to keep it.

When I ran races with my dad, sometimes his hand would be on my back pushing me up hills when I needed it. Now whenever I need momentum, all I have to do is think back to how it felt to have his hand pushing me up that hill—and I can tap into that momentum and use it in other parts of my life.

That's what momentum is: it's like a hand on your back that helps you along and makes things require less effort. Whenever there's anything in your life that makes things easier—anything that helps you go even further than you ever expected—you need to tap into it and understand what it is. It's about recognizing momentum, what's bringing that momentum, and then trying your best to both appreciate it and keep it going.

For example, maybe you chose versions of exercises in your workout that you like, and not only did your body respond to them, but the exercise made you enjoy the process even more. Or maybe there's a new friend or a group of people you're hanging out with, and they're bringing joy into your life that is helping you get more from the program. Or perhaps just getting up fifteen minutes earlier on certain days made sticking with the program much easier to do.

The point is, can you stop for long enough to realize what momentum looks like outside of just physically feeling it, so can you do your best to recreate it? Because some people look at these gifts when they're given to them and either don't appreciate them in the moment, fail to take advantage of them, or fail to notice them entirely. And when you do that, you remain still.

That won't be you. So find those moments of momentum, be thankful for those gifts, do your best to make the most of them, and try your hardest to earn momentum the next time through.

LIFT Your Goals Further

The first thing I would always do as an athlete when starting a new season is reevaluate and reset—if necessary—both my process and outcome goals. That's when I would ask myself whether I had the right goals in place: Did I think through my goals in the right way, and did I assume too much too early?

Now, it's your turn.

Outcome Goals

Having outcome goals in place should have helped you measure the success of the LIFTED program as you use it. At the end of four weeks:

> Ask yourself, Am I any closer to any goal? If so, great job! And know that the longer you stay with the program, the closer you'll come next time. So

if you can say with complete certainty that you're a little closer now than you were four weeks ago and that you're still passionate about your goal, then keep it for the next time through.

If you did manage to hit a goal, ask yourself, *Is there any way to change this goal to go a little further?* For example, maybe one of your process goals was to eat healthy at least five days a week, but you can always do six or seven. Or maybe one of your outcome goals was to lose five pounds, but you still have thirty more to go. Now's the time to change your goals to reflect the next personal mountain to climb.

If you didn't reach a goal, be honest and ask yourself, *Did I bite off a little more than I could chew?* If so, then that's okay. Using the same examples I just mentioned, if your goal was to eat healthy five days a week but you ate healthy for only three, give yourself credit. If your goal was to lose five pounds but you lost only three, give yourself credit. Then use what you now know about yourself to create a new, more attainable goal. So maybe the next time around your goals might be to eat healthy four days a week or lose another three pounds. The more manageable you make your goals, the more you'll manage to reach them.

LIFT Your Dream Board Higher

Obviously there will be some big dreams on that Dream Board that didn't come true in just four weeks, and that's fine. Just remember, that wasn't the purpose of putting them up there. I still have dreams on my Dream Board that have been up there for years. This has all been about getting you to face your dreams each and every day, not about achieving them within a certain amount of time.

This is the time when I want you to step back and look at the entire Dream Board. Now, instead of it serving as a reminder of your dreams, I want you to focus on your Dream Board to see whether there's anything you need to change or rearrange on it.

You may find yourself in an entirely different headspace now in as little as four weeks. You may look up at your Dream Board now and see things you wish to change. That's the beautiful thing about a program that affects so many parts of your life:

You're going to see changes in yourself that aren't solely physical. You're going to see changes in the things you want. You're going to see changes in the things you aspire to be.

I found that the best way to rethink your Dream Board is to ask yourself the following questions:

Are there any dreams I managed to achieve?

If the answer is yes, I'm so proud of you! You can choose to take it down or do what I do with certain dreams and keep that dream up there as a reminder of what's possible. It's like a trophy! Let it be an example to you each and every day of what you're capable of so that if you ever doubt you can achieve any other dreams on your Dream Board, you can look at that one and realize that once, that was merely a dream as well—and you made that dream come true.

Something I'll never take down? I'm with Nike now, but I put a Nike swoosh on my Dream Board a long time before that. I had always dreamt of becoming a Nike-sponsored athlete. Just watching Nike commercials as a kid and seeing all their athletes, I used to think, *Oh man—to be a Nike athlete!* So when I actually became a Nike trainer, it was one of my biggest dreams come true. That swoosh is still up there on my Dream Board. I still get butterflies every time I see it because I had put it up there before it happened, and I'm so proud of it that I'll never take it down—*ever*.

Are there any dreams
I want to put closer in the center?

As I mentioned at the beginning of this book, I like to put the dreams that mean the most to me dead center in my Dream Board. You may have a different system in place. No matter how you arrange it, now is the time to look at all your dreams and see whether certain dreams mean more to you now than others. And if any have changed priority, move them around your Dream Board so they're located in whatever spot they should be. However, if where your dreams are arranged doesn't matter to you, that's fine too. You can leave everything right where it is. Think about it like rearranging the furniture in your room—sometimes it helps to freshen things up!

Are there any dreams
I no longer wish to dream?

Something that most people don't expect to happen when they start LIFTING themselves for the first time is how it changes your perspective. Suddenly you may find that certain things you *thought* were important aren't important at all or not as important as you thought they were.

Dreams change, especially as we become more enlightened to what really matters in life. So don't be surprised if you see a dream up there that's no longer a dream. And if you do—if your heart, soul, and very being are no longer vested in that dream—you can take it down. There's no failure in that. In fact, it just leaves a space open for another dream that may make even more of an impact in your life.

Are there any new dreams I need to add?

I find that a lot of people discover dreams inside themselves that they didn't know they had once their mind, body, and spirit are more in tune with one another. And maybe that's you. Maybe you didn't dream as big at the beginning of the program, but now you're dreaming even bigger than before. Or maybe certain dreams didn't seem possible. But seeing how you've moved the needle forward on the rest of the dreams on your Dream Board, you're now more dialed into what's possible. So get them up there!

Final point: Just because I've asked you to reset your Dream Board before restarting the program, that doesn't mean you can't do it at any time during the program. They're *your* dreams—I just want to make sure they aren't just sitting in front of you but instead always moving forward.

LIFT Your Mind Even Higher

After four weeks the thing I always have clients do when it comes to their mind is to be honest. I know I said this earlier, and I want you to be honest about every portion of the program, but when it comes to meditation, there are some that don't take it as seriously as others.

Maybe you picked this book up entirely because you were interested in just changing your body. Maybe the whole meditation portion was something you didn't expect to see. So ask yourself, Have you really been doing it every day? Did you do it only during the workout portion? Did you actually skip doing it during the workout portion just to make the routine go faster?

Ready for some honesty? I'll admit it: this is my book. But a week might go by, and I'll realize that I didn't meditate for a few days. I'm not perfect, and neither are you, and that's entirely okay. That's why my first tip to taking your mind to a different level is,

Make Your Mind a Priority: When I have to get real with myself because I've let meditation slip out of my daily routine from time to time, I make sure I start my day by meditating before I do anything else. I know I told you that before, and I also said you had options. But if you're real with yourself and admit that you weren't doing it on a regular basis, now's the time to make it a morning ritual so you're less likely to neglect it.

Expand Your Mind Exponentially: If you did meditate every day, that means you've already begun to notice a difference. So do yourself a favor and see what else is out there!

The type of meditation I've asked you to do is known as mindfulness meditation, where you're not focused on any particular thing; instead, you just observe all of your thoughts and senses without attaching to them or judging them.

But there are other types of meditation. One type requires enhanced concentration on one specific thing for the entire time, otherwise known as *focused attention* meditation. There is also *effortless transcending* meditation, where the goal is to create a state of nothingness by making your mind become a blank slate.

With so many options out there, what you choose to try is entirely up to you. Personally, I go to a meditation center when I can because it's a very different experience to go someplace for thirty minutes where someone guides you through the meditation. There's a peaceful energy in places like that, even if it's just one time per month. I also know that once the door closes and the meditation starts, I can't leave! When I have trouble being disciplined, I need some help!

But that's me! Do your mind a favor—and your body and spirit as well—and explore beyond what I've shown you. Now that you got the hang of it, try whatever may be waiting for your mind to find.

Reflect on Each Week and Every Day: Living in New York City, I have the opportunity to be annoyed, agitated, and irritated at every moment of the day. But when I meditate, there is a calmness about me. When I walk outside after class it almost feels as if I am floating. Tourists may walk slowly in front of me, a biker might cut me off, and someone could be laying on their horn a block away. And at that moment, if I allow myself to pay attention to it, I'll accept it as part of my moment, let it go, and be unfazed by it. But I also know of plenty of times when I'm not in that mindset, and every little thing builds up and creates more stress.

That's why after a month of meditation I think it's important to realize the impact it's made on your decisions. Try to think back on specific stressful days when you either kept your cool or perhaps didn't handle things as well as you could have.

If you meditated on those days, did you notice a difference? Did you handle any situation better than you might have otherwise? Were there any days when you felt proud of yourself because you remained calm and less anxious? Or perhaps a friend, family member, or coworker complimented you for tackling something better than expected? On the flip side, were there any days when you felt extremely stressed, and did that day happen to be one when you chose not to meditate?

What I'd like you to do, if possible, is try to make a connection between meditation and the moods you may have had during certain situations. That's the most exciting part about meditation—that's the insightful, powerful part: when you can reflect on things that worked or when you're actually noticing them happening at that moment. That first time when, for example, someone might yell at you for some reason and you realize, *I'm not being reactive . . . and I can deal with this.* And you do—with a cooler head and an open heart.

Sometimes it takes reminding ourselves how meditation is working behind the scenes throughout the day to keep us more positive and calm. Very soon you'll begin to see parallels and connections between how you handle things that are intense or stressful and how often you meditate. And the more connections you see, the more meditation will become an even more important part of your day.

Shoot for More Time and Space: By the end of the program you'll have performed a minimum of thirteen minutes of meditation a day. That's why, if you're starting the program again, I'd like you to start Day One doing fourteen minutes a day, then see if you can increase it by one minute per week. As you repeat the program over and over again, just start where you left off and add one minute each week. Eventually you'll find the sweet spot of how much time you have to meditate, but ideally, if you reach thirty minutes after a few times, that's fantastic!

Another way to make the most out of your meditation is to try to create even more space between your thoughts. When you first started LIFTED you may have found that the best you were able to do was put a couple of seconds between each thought. So this time through, take notice of those spaces and see whether they lengthen at all.

But wait: I don't want you focusing on the space between your thoughts *while* you meditate; instead, just take a moment afterward to reflect on the growing space. It will naturally happen, I promise you. And as you grow to have more space between your thoughts, you'll also be training yourself to have more space between moments of reaction.

LIFT Your Body Even Higher

The beauty of the Body portion of LIFTED is that there's plenty of room to grow. You can always stick with the way you originally performed each move, and you'll still see your body change as a result. But if you're looking for a little more of a challenge, you can try a more advanced version of any or all of the exercises in the program.

So if you needed to step into the program using the easiest versions of most or all of the moves, try to perform a few exercises as they were originally described. If you did the program as described, then try some of the more advanced exercises on for size.

Unleash the Outline— But Only When You're Ready

Once you reach a place where the routine is less of a challenge and you can do the more advanced versions of all the exercises, you have the power to make your own LIFTED routine.

That's right! What I've given you is the outline of the workout, and now you get to create your own, using the exercises you already know. You see, each exercise falls into one of three categories: an upper body/total body exercise, a lower-body exercise, and a core exercise. Here's where each exercise ranks:

LB (LOWER BODY)

- squats
- reverse lunges
- drop squats
- wall sits
- single leg Romanian deadlifts
- fast feet
- speed skaters
- high knee sprints
- plyo side lunge

UB/TB (UPPER BODY/TOTAL BODY)

- push-ups
- renegade row
- dips
- burpees
- mountain climbers
- sumo squat fighter

CORE

- planks
- side planks
- Russian twists
- goddess sit-ups
- bird dogs
- v-ups
- glute bridges
- slow bicycles
- high planks with shoulder tap
- up-down planks
- rockstars
- reach backs

So to create your own workout, here's what you'll do:

- Start with five minutes of meditation.
- Do a Dynamic Warm-Up.
- Next, take one exercise from each category, and design your own three-move complex. First, grab an LB move, then a UB/TB move, then a CORE move. Got your three-move circuit? Great—now make another one, only pick a different LB, UB/TB, and CORE move. Now you should have two complexes, creating one six-move circuit! Do each exercise for one straight minute, one after the other without resting, then rest one full minute. Repeat the six-move circuit for a total of three to four rounds.
- Do five more minutes of meditation.
- Run through your six-move circuit one final time. Do each move for one straight minute, one after the other, without rest.

Finish your session with a five-minute Bottle It Up!

By the way, do you always have to take things to the next level with exercise? Not all the time, no. Whatever you do, I don't want you to feel any pressure to create your own workouts immediately. This is only for when your body is ready to move past what I've already shown you. That might happen the second time around if you're already fit. That might happen in six months, or maybe years from now.

If you're happy with the way the program is working in its original format, just keep doing it. As I've said, everyone's body is different, and so long as what you're doing is LIFTING you upward, that's what matters. You need to understand that when that time comes, know that your body has been progressing the entire time. You've continuously been LIFTING up your body throughout those weeks, months, or even years—and that's what it's all about.

But know this: if you stick with the same workout repeatedly without tweaking or changing it, your body eventually adapts and becomes more efficient at doing it. That may sound amazing, but it's not.

The more efficient your body becomes with a program, the fewer calories and less lean muscle you'll build as you use it that program. You need to think of exercise having an expiration date! After four weeks that time is usually up.

The good news: by mixing things up slightly in your routine, even if it's just re-arranging the order of your exercises, you can keep your muscles guessing and your body out of its comfort zone. You'll be forcing it to constantly be ready for anything and, as a result, continuously building lean muscle and burning calories.

LIFT Your Spirit Even Higher

For four weeks straight I asked you to try a variety of different things each week meant to LIFT your spirit in various ways. By the end of the journey, hopefully, you were able to do all of them. But even if you just did one or two, you still managed to LIFT your spirit along the way—and I'm proud of you. And you should be proud of yourself too.

If it's your first time through LIFTED, I'm sure there were a few parts you didn't get around to doing. Maybe it was because you couldn't think of anything or anyone who fit that situation. Maybe you weren't able to tackle certain tasks because you were just starting out the program and wanted to get your feet wet first. All of that is okay by me. Now, here's what you can do the next time that can elevate your spirit even further.

Focus On What Fell Behind: Your next time through, if there were any spirit-lifting tactics you hadn't tried, try to make those your top priority. But if for some reason that's not possible, ask yourself why: Are you too afraid? Am I asking you to do something you're not ready to do? Or do you just not know where to begin? Whatever the reason, think about how you can overcome that obstacle so you can give that tactic a try.

Remember Which Lifted You the Most: Take a look through all the tactics you tried in order to raise your spirit during those four weeks, and flag which ones brought you the most happiness. I personally guarantee that if you tried more than one, they didn't all LIFT your spirits equally. You'll know which ones had the most effect in a positive way in your life, so make sure you do your best to repeat whichever ones had the greatest influence on your spirit.

Rinse, Repeat, Rejuvenate! The beauty of the Spirit section of LIFTED is that you can do all of it over and over and over again. There isn't such a thing as overtraining your spirit. So even if you managed to do all eighteen in four weeks—and if you did, that's incredible—then do it all over again. Each of those tactics can be used with

Push Yourself—But Know Your Limits

As much as I want you to continue advancing the program, I also want you to listen to your mind, body, and spirit to make sure you never push yourself harder than what is healthy for you.

About five or six years ago I was teaching spin, running more classes, and I was getting super-lean. I was eating right, lifting a lot, and feeling great. It was a very momentous part of my career because I felt amazing and was in my most Type A groove. There was no stopping me, and I felt I couldn't afford to slow down.

But if anybody should understand being in tune with how your body feels when you're overusing it, it's me because plantar fasciitis ended my basketball career early. So when I began to feel this little thing in my foot again, I should've stopped and had it checked out, but I kept going. I wasn't resting enough and hadn't been practicing what I was preaching. Training had become my second career after basketball ended, so I continued to push myself to the limit.

Then I was at a pride parade, just hanging out with friends and skipping down the street . . . when I heard a pop. I had torn my gastrocnemius muscle—a fancy name for the calf muscle in the back of your lower leg.

Just skipping.

It was a very similar injury to what I had done in basketball. When I tore my fascia playing basketball, I heard a familiar pop in the back of my foot back then too. So that day on the street I thought to myself, *What are you doing, Holly? Here we go again.*

The truth is that when you don't learn lessons in life, life dishes them out again. I think life decided to wake me up a little bit that day. Luckily I was out of work for only a couple of weeks at most, but it reminded me that I was far from invincible. The exact same mistake that brought my basketball career to a halt—and I did it again.

So if at any point you feel you're pushing yourself too hard, I want you to take that moment to pause. Know that if you choose to stop LIFTING yourself at any point, you won't immediately fall back down to earth. This is a journey with many hills and valleys, ups and downs, and, sometimes, a handful of pit stops. So listen to yourself, believe what you're telling yourself, and always keep a pace you can handle for the long haul.

This isn't a sprint.

It's a journey.

One that will last a lifetime—if you allow it to.

different people and different situations, making it impossible not to be able to do them on a continual basis. So go ahead—your spirit is waiting!

LIFT Your Fuel Even Higher

Remember that food journal I asked you to keep? The one where I asked you to write down everything you ate, including the time and the emotion you felt when you were eating it?

Your first time through LIFTED I just wanted you to go through the process. I didn't want you to think too hard. I didn't want you to become too introspective about what you ate—yet. But now, if you're looking to get more from the program, it's time to look at what you've written to see what you could work on.

Look Back for Patterns: I want you to go back and look at the big picture—those big-picture answers are there. You know which steps made easier to eat healthier and which mistakes you made that messed up what you meant to eat for the day. Once you begin to recognize certain patterns, you can begin to strategize around any areas of weakness you might come across as well as encourage anything that might've helped you eat healthier throughout the day.

One way that I find that clients figure out those patterns faster is by asking the following questions:

What held me back? For me, I've come to know over the years that it's not a good idea for me to buy jars of almond butter or big tubs of cashews because I'll eat the entire thing. I mean all of it—sometimes in just one sitting.

But if I buy almonds in bulk, I won't. For some reason I have the willpower to stop at a handful, which is why I choose to keep those around more often than almond butter and cashews, even though all three provide the same nutritional value.

Now it's your turn. Focus on the bad decisions you may have made, and ask yourself what triggered it those times when you chose to eat poorly. Maybe when you're eating out, the meal you chose that came out of the kitchen was a little bigger than you expected. Maybe you've noticed that every day at three o'clock after you check your emails you eat a candy bar or something else unhealthy. Maybe instead of going out for coffee with your friends, you chose to go out for dessert instead. Maybe you went food shopping on an empty stomach and ended up buying more junk food than you normally would.

If you look hard enough, you may have created situations that tested the boundaries of your willpower. And with just a little tweaking, you can prevent those situations from happening again or recognize how, in those situations, you can make smarter choices next time.

Was I hungry for the right reasons? I hope that as you look through your journal you see nothing but a whole bunch of H's—that every time you ate, you were hungry. But if you're human—and I know I am—there are probably a few other letters in that journal as well.

Now is the time to tally up all those letters. That's right: add them up and see which is higher. You may notice a trend in how often you eat when you're emotional or that the only times you ever seem to eat badly are when you're out with your friends and being social. You may discover that you eat more out of boredom than you do out of hunger.

You'll be surprised at how tallying up these letters can give you a quick, broad overview of what might be behind what's holding you back nutritionally. And with that information, you can lay out a better game plan to prevent it from happening next time.

For example, if you predominately eat out of boredom, now you know you need to find other things to keep your mind occupied. If you tend to eat a lot socially, you may need to think ahead about which events you attend or plan ahead to know before you get there what to avoid.

Think about it this way: the more H's you see, the more Holly will be cheering for you!

What helped me out? Remember what I said about momentum? Maybe you've noticed that on days when you wake up early you made smarter choices. Maybe preparing healthier meals earlier in the week and putting them in the freezer helped you eat like a rock star for the entire week. If you see certain decisions that helped you make smarter nutritional choices, then it's time to double down on those decisions and make them a bigger part of your routine. Remember: this program is about *life*—this is your new *life*!

Afterword

When I was in college my strength and conditioning coach, Greg Werner, was my mentor, and to this day he has always been such a rock in my career. When I was super-lost after leaving pro basketball and wasn't sure how I would carve out my place in the fitness world, the most powerful thing he said to me was

The seeds of greatness are planted deep inside you, Holly. But they will only grow fully when you share them with others.

At that moment, when I couldn't find the strength to LIFT myself, it dawned on me that when you start to give back to people, that's when you "close the circle." I finally understood that when you can see the difference you're making in other people's lives, that's when you'll feel completely fulfilled.

That's what LIFTED has become for me. Through my classes and now with this book, I feel there's a part of me that's finally closing the circle. And so far what my coach said about feeling completely fulfilled is coming true.

So . . . who can you share this program with? Who in your life right now is struggling? Who do you think in your life right now could use a little more joy? Who do you know right now who needs a little LIFT? Could you share this program with them? Could they become a new workout partner who might even help LIFT you a little higher?

The point is that can you give back to someone else and spread the love. If you've genuinely experienced the difference LIFTED has made in your life, wouldn't you want to share that with someone?

When someone takes this path with you, it not only makes the journey a little less difficult; it makes it more joyous as well. Because you'll have somebody who understands what you're experiencing—someone who can be a "hand on your back" when you need momentum, just as you can be theirs. You'll be rising together, and you get to know what I feel every single day I teach.

I'm a leader. I'm a dealer in hope. I'm brave with my life so that others will be brave with theirs.

Now, it's *your* turn to close your circle—and LIFT your life to a place you never thought possible. So make yourself proud today!

Acknowledgments

Mom and Dad: You have been with me for every twist and turn. The sacrifices you made as parents I can now appreciate. You supported me through the entire journey. You drove miles. Spent money. You were my greatest cheerleaders. You continue to be my greatest teachers.

My siblings: Bryan, John, and Sarah Rilinger, thank you for your undying support. Countless games and road trips. I can still see you there cheering me on. I know at times growing up it must have felt like the "Holly Show."

My grandparents: For providing a solid midwestern upbringing. Milking the cows included. Grandma, I hated it for years but thank you for my strong legs.

Greg Werner: For being my greatest mentor. I turn to you when I cannot find the words to motivate and inspire myself.

My literary agents, Jeff Googel and Eve Atterman.

Doug Scott: Boy, did you intimidate me that first day I met you. Thank you for believing in me. Thank you for your mentorship and your friendship. "Oh the places you'll go."

Lisette Sand-Freedman and Brad Z: For helping me reach the next level. Am I there?

Myatt Murphy (of course): For helping me bring my thoughts to life—we make a great team.

Carolyn Brown: Thank you for being my "go-to" on nutrition and spreading your deliciousness all over the world.

Sonni Tallant: Thank you for looking me in the eyes, shaking my hand, and believing in a stranger after UPW many years ago. You helped me take my first steps and have been there for the entire journey.

Lisa Curtis: For helping me shed a layer and awakening my spirit. We will always have something special.

Sam Manheimer: For sticking with me through thick and thin. You deserve a medal.

Flywheel: For providing a platform for growth. Specifically Ruth Zukerman and Jay Galluzo. The infamous chair hug will live on forever.

My Loyal Flywheel Riders: You gave me life every day for the past six years. It's me and you—you and me. A few front-row shout-outs: Clem, Amanda, Jenny D, CY Eats, Tania, Liz, Leslie, Leah, G$, Eric, Anita, Lisa, and Andrew.

My greatest support group. My close friends who have seen me through the ups and downs—your support is what has kept my fire burning bright.

Nike: For helping a childhood dream come to life.

LL: Thanks for LIFTED and many other things.

Patty LaRocco: You showed me New York.

Dan Feldman: It's people like you who spin dreams into motion. You offered me your help when I was basically a stranger outside that spin room.

Bob Difazio: Thank you for your guidance.

Norma Jean Callahan: For seeing a girl in need, helping me find my light, and rescuing me.

Toni Haber: For giving me that Tony Robbins ticket.

Frieda Max: For letting me sleep on your sofa when I ran out of money at the beginning of this journey.

Laura Scott: You picked me up off the ground of NYC and gave me hope.

Paola de Telig: Thank you for opening my spirit and mind to the gift of meditation.

Jay Rather: For the safety net you dropped, allowing me to move to NYC.

Sarah Gillespie: For helping me pick up furniture off the streets of NYC and lighting that spark.

Besty Blose: For countless rebounds and many other things.

My basketball coaches over the years: For helping mold me into the person I am today.

Susie: For helping me grow.

Notes

Chapter 1

1. Aymeric Guillot, Kevin Moschberger, and Christian Collet, "Coupling Movement with Imagery as a New Perspective for Motor Imagery Practice: A Within-Subjects Design," *Behavioral and Brain Functions* 9, no. 8 (February 2013).

2. Andrew M. Lane, Peter Totterdell, Ian MacDonald, Tracey J. Devonport, Andrew P. Friesen, Christopher J. Beedie et al., "Brief Online Training Enhances Competitive Performance: Findings of the BBC Lab UK Psychological Skills Intervention Study," *Frontiers in Psychology* 7 (2016): 413.

Chapter 2

1. Tonya L. Jacobs, Elissa S. Epel, Jue Lin, Elizabeth H. Blackburn, Owen M. Wolkowitz, David A. Bridwell, Anthony P. Zanesco, et al., "Intensive Meditation Training, Immune Cell Telomerase Activity, and Psychological Mediators," *Psychoneuroendocrinology* 36, no. 5 (June 2011): 664–681.

2. J. C. Ong, R. Manber, Z. Segal, Y. Xia, S. Shapiro, and J. K. Wyatt, "A Randomized Controlled Trial of Mindfulness Meditation for Chronic Insomnia," *Sleep* 37, no. 9 (September 2014): 1553–1563.

3. Prashant Kaul, Jason Passafiume, R. Craig Sargent, and Bruce F. O'Hara, "Meditation Acutely Improves Psychomotor Vigilance, and May Decrease Sleep Need," *Behavioral and Brain Functions* 6, no. 1 (July 2010): 1–9.

4. Y. Y. Tang, Q. Lu, M. Fan, Y. Yang, and M. I. Posner, "Mechanisms of White Matter Changes Induced by Meditation," *Proceedings of the National Academy of Sciences of the United States* 109, no. 26 (June 2012): 10570–10574.

5. A. B. Newberg, N. Wintering, H. Roggenkampa, D. S. Khalsa, M. R. Waldman, and K. Thakur, "Meditation Effects on Cognitive Function and Cerebral Blood Flow in Subjects with Memory Loss: A Preliminary Study," *Journal of Alzheimer's Disease* 20, no. 2 (2010): 517–526; A. Mohan, R. Sharma, and R. L. Bijlani, "Effect of Meditation on Stress-Induced Changes in Cognitive Functions," *Journal of Alternative and Complementary Medicine* 17, no. 3 (March 2011): 207–212; O. Singleton, M. Vangel, S. W. Lazar, B. K. Holzel, N. Brach, and

J. Carmody, "Change in Brainstem Gray Matter Concentration Following a Mindfulness-Based Intervention is Correlated with Improvement in Psychological Well-Being," *Frontiers in Human Neuroscience* 8, no. 1 (February 2014): 33.

6. Y. Singh, R. Sharma, and A. Talwar, "Immediate and Long-Term Effects of Meditation on Acute Stress Reactivity, Cognitive Functions, and Intelligence," *Alternative Therapies in Health and Medicine* 18, no. 6 (November–December 2012): 46–53.

7. Manoj K. Bhasin, Jeffrey A. Dusek, Bei-Hung Chang, Marie G. Joseph, John W. Denninger, Gregory L. Fricchione, Herbert Benson, et al., "Relaxation Response Induces Temporal Transcriptome Changes in Energy Metabolism, Insulin Secretion, and Inflammatory Pathways," *PLoS One* 8, no. 5 (May 2013): e62817.

8. Peter la Cour and Marian Petersen, "Effects of Mindfulness Meditation on Chronic Pain: A Randomized Controlled Trial," *Pain Medicine* 16, no. 4 (April 2015): 641–652.

9. Shawn N. Katterman, Brighid M. Kleinman, Megan M. Hood, Lisa M. Nackers, and Joyce A. Corsica, "Mindfulness Meditation as an Intervention for Binge Eating, Emotional Eating, and Weight Loss: A Systematic Review," *Eating Behaviors* 15, no. 2 (April 2014): 197–204.

10. Márcia de Fátima Rosas Marchiori, Elisa Harumi Kozasa, Roberto Dischinger Miranda, André Luiz Monezi Andrade, Tatiana Caccese Perrotti, and José Roberto Leite, "Decrease in Blood Pressure and Improved Psychological Aspects Through Meditation Training in Hypertensive Older Adults: A Randomized Control Study," *Geriatrics and Gerontology International* 15, no. 10 (October 2015): 1158–1164; J. W. Anderson, C. Liu, and R. J. Kryscio, "Blood Pressure Response to Transcendental Meditation: A Meta-Analysis," *American Journal of Hypertension* 21, no. 3 (March 2008): 310–316.

Chapter 3

1. Physical Activity, CDC, www.cdc.gov/physicalactivity/growingstronger/why.

Chapter 4

1. M. E. Seligman, T. A. Steen, N. Park, and C. Peterson, "Positive Psychology Progress: Empirical Validation of Interventions," *American Psychologist* 60, no. 1 (July–August 2005): 410–421.

2. R. A. Emmons and M. E. McCullough, "Counting Blessings Versus Burdens: An Experimental Investigation of Gratitude and Subjective Well-Being in Daily Life," *Journal of Personality and Social Psychology* 84, no. 2 (February 2003): 377–389.

3. Lung Hung Chen and Chia-Huei Wu, "Gratitude Enhances Change in Athletes' Self-Esteem: The Moderating Role of Trust in Coach," *Journal of Applied Sport Psychology* 26, no. 3 (2014): 349–362.

4. N. M. Lambert and F. D. Fincham, "Expressing Gratitude to a Partner Leads to More Relationship Maintenance Behavior," *Emotion* 11, no. 1 (February 2011): 52–60.

5. Alex M. Wood, Stephen Joseph, Joanna Lloyd, and Samuel Atkins, "Gratitude Influences Sleep Through the Mechanism of Pre-Sleep Cognitions," *Journal of Psychosomatic Research* 66, no. 1 (January 2009): 43–48.

6. Jo-Ann Tsang, Thomas P. Carpenter, James A. Roberts, Michael B. Frisch, and Robert D. Carlisle, "Why Are Materialists Less Happy? The Role of Gratitude and Need Satisfaction in the Relationship Between Materialism and Life Satisfaction," *Personality and Individual Differences* 64 (2014): 62–66.

7. E. Kross, M. G. Berman, W. Mischel, E. E. Smith, and T. D. Wager, "Social Rejection Shares Somatosensory Representations with Physical Pain," *Proceedings of the National Academy of the Sciences of the United States* 108, no. 15 (April 2011): 6270–6275.

Chapter 6

1. Angela Kong, Shirley A. A. Beresford, Catherine M. Alfano, Karen E. Foster-Schubert, Marian L. Neuhouser, Donna B. Johnson, Catherine Duggan, et al., "Self-Monitoring and Eating-Related Behaviors Are Associated with 12-Month Weight Loss in Postmenopausal Overweight-to-Obese Women," *Journal of the Academy of Nutrition and Dietetics* 112, no. 9 (September 2012): 1428–1435.

2. Laruette Dubé, Patrick Webb, Narendra K. Arora, Prabhu Pingalid, Peter Helfer, and Thomas R. Shultz, "The Effects of Nutrition Labeling on Consumer Food Choice: A Psychological Experiment and Computational Model," *Annals of the New York Academy of Sciences* 1331 (December 2014): 174–185.

3. J. M. Poti, M. A. Mendez, S. W. Ng, and B. M. Popkin, "Is the Degree of Food Processing and Convenience Linked with the Nutritional Quality of Foods Purchased by US Households?" *American Journal of Clinical Nutrition* 101, no. 6 (June 2015): 1251–1262.

4. Josh West, "Pilot Test of a Bites-Focused Weight Loss Intervention," *Advances in Obesity, Weight Management and Control* 3, no. 1 (October 2015).

5. X. Wang, Y. Ouyang, J. Liu, M. Zhu, G. Zhao, W. Bao, and F. B. Hu. "Fruit and Vegetable Consumption and Mortality from All Causes, Cardiovascular Disease, and Cancer: Systematic Review and Dose-Response Meta-Analysis of Prospective Cohort Studies," *BMJ* 349 (July 2014): g4490.

6. UY. T. Lo, Y. H. Chang, M. L. Wahlqvist, H. B. Huang, and M. S. Lee, "Spending on Vegetable and Fruit Consumption Could Reduce All-Cause Mortality Among Older Adults," *Nutrition Journal* 11 (2012): 113.

7. A. Bellavia, S. C. Larsson, M. Bottai, A. Wolk, and N. Orsini, "Fruit and Vegetable Consumption and All-Cause Mortality: A Dose-Response Analysis," *American Journal of Clinical Nutrition* 98, no. 2 (August 2013): 454–459.

8. F. Imamura, R. Micah, J. H. Wu, Otto M. C. de Oliveira, F. O. Otite, A. I. Abioye, and D. Mozaffarian, "Effects of Saturated Fat, Polyunsaturated Fat, Monounsaturated Fat, and Carbohydrate on Glucose-Insulin Homeostasis: A Systematic Review and Meta-analysis of Randomised Controlled Feeding Trials," *PLoS Medicine* 13, no. 7 (July 2016): e1002087.

9. K. J. Navara, and S. E. Pinson, "Yolk and Albumen Corticosterone Concentrations in Eggs Laid by White Versus Brown Caged Laying Hens," *Poultry Science* 89, no. 7 (July 2010): 1509–1513.

10. Qiao-Ping Wang, Yong Qi Lin, Lei Zhang, Yana A. Wilson, Lisa J. Oyston, James Cotterell, Yue Qi, et al., "Sucralose Promotes Food Intake Through NPY and a Neuronal Fasting Response," *Cell Metabolism* 24, no. 1 (July 2016): 75–90.

11. David Zeevi, Tal Korem, Niv Zmora, David Israeli, Daphna Rothschild, Adina Weinberger, Orly Ben-Yacov, et al., "Personalized Nutrition by Prediction of Glycemic Responses," *Cell* 163, no. 5 (November 2015): 1079–1094.

12. K. J. Duffey and J. Poti, "Modeling the Effect of Replacing Sugar-Sweetened Beverage Consumption with Water on Energy Intake, HBI Score, and Obesity Prevalence," *Nutrients* 8, no. 7 (June 2016): E395.

13. T. S. Conner, K. L. Brookie, A. C. Richardson, and M. A. Polak, "On Carrots and Curiosity: Eating Fruit and Vegetables Is Associated with Greater Flourishing in Daily Life," *British Journal of Health Psychology* 20, no. 2 (May 2015): 413–427.

Index

breakfast
    Awesome Avo-Baked-Eggs, 173
    Excellent Avocado Sweet Potato "Toast,"
       175
    Fantastic Herb Frittata, 174
    Zap Your Appetite Smoothie, 175
    Zesty Coconut Parfait, 174
breathing
    and controlling anger, 126–27
    in meditation, 37–38
Brown, Carolyn, 168
burpees, 78–79
business cards, 16
butt kicks, 64

C

calories, versus ingredients, 156–57
carbohydrates, 157–58
cardio day, 55
carrots
    Miso Happy Salad, 177
    Spicy Thai Carrot Noodles, 183
chest stretch, 106
chicken
    ABC De-licious Salad (Avocado-
      Basil-Chicken), 176
    Chicken Lettuce "Mock-o Tacos,"
      179–80
    Pistachi-Oh-Yes! Crusted Chicken,
      184
Chicken Lettuce "Mock-o Tacos," 179–80
Choco-Espresso Protein Smoothie, 186
clothing
    for meditation, 33–34
    for working out, 49
cobra, 105

coconut
    Zesty Coconut Parfait, 174
coconut milk
    Zap Your Appetite Smoothie, 175
coffee
    Choco-Espresso Protein Smoothie, 186
comfort zone, stepping outside of, 120
commitments, dropping, 133–34
cooldown, 52–53
    chest stretch, 106
    cobra, 105
    hurdler stretch, 103
    quadriceps stretch, 104
    seated glute stretch, 107

D

dancing, 68
decisions, meditation's effect on, 28–29
depression, 118, 132
diet. *See* eating; food; nutrition
dinner
    Pistachi-Oh-Yes! Crusted Chicken,
      184
    Savory Pesto Turkey Sliders Over
      Greens, 183
    Simply Succulent Zucchini Soup, 182
    Spicy Secret Weapon Salmon, 181
    Spicy Thai Carrot Noodles, 183
dips, 80
Dream Board, 12–18, 192–94
drop squats, 97

E

eating. *See also* food; nutrition
    benefits of healthy, 166–67
    boredom in, 168

S

salads
 ABC De-licious Salad (Avocado-Basil-Chicken), 176
 Miso Happy Salad, 177
salmon
 Miso Happy Salad, 177
 Spicy Secret Weapon Salmon, 181
saturated fats, 158–59
Savory Pesto Turkey Sliders Over Greens, 183
seated glute stretch, 107
self-compassion, 128
self-esteem, gratitude and, 121
shaking things up, 117
shoes, for working out, 49
Shrimp, Simple Lemon-Basil, 177–78
side lunge, 66
side plank, 75
Simple Lemon-Basil Shrimp, 177–78
Simply Succulent Zucchini Soup, 182
single-leg Romanian deadlifts, 90
sit-ups, goddess, 86
skin, 167
skipping in place, 67
sleep, 27
slow bicycles, 94
small victories, celebrating, 123–24
smoothies, 166
 Choco-Espresso Protein Smoothie, 186
 Zap Your Appetite Smoothie, 175

snacks, 164
 Apple-Almond Butter Rings, 185
 Choco-Espresso Protein Smoothie, 186
 Turkey Rev-Up Roll-Ups, 186
snowboarding injury, 130–32
sounds, in meditation, 38–39
speed skaters, 85
Spicy Secret Weapon Salmon, 181
Spicy Thai Carrot Noodles, 183
spirit, 129–35
 bottling up, 148
 cutting things out to strengthen, 129–35
 eating to please, 163
 engaging, 19–20
 lifting, 111–13, 200–202
 location of, 114
 owning, 121–25
 person supporting, 115
 seeking, 116–20
 soundtrack for, 114–15
 understanding, 126–29
Spirit Soundtrack, 114–15
Spotify, 108
squats, 72
 drop squats, 97
 sumo squat fighter, 98–99
strength training, importance of, 109. *See also* main exercises
stretches
 chest stretch, 106
 cobra, 105
 hurdler stretch, 103
 quadriceps stretch, 104
 seated glute stretch, 107

Z